A Nurse's Guide to
Implementing Self-Care

# HELP
# YOURSELF...

## Dr. Lillian Gonzalez

First published by Ultimate World Publishing 2019
Copyright © 2019 Dr. Lillian Gonzalez

ISBN

Paperback: 978-1-925884-61-6
eBook: 978-1-925884-62-3

**Cover design:** Ultimate World Publishing
**Layout and typesetting:** Ultimate World Publishing
**Editor:** Marinda Wilkinson

ULTIMATE WORLD
——— PUBLISHING ———

Ultimate World Publishing
Diamond Creek,
Victoria Australia 3089
www.writeabook.com.au

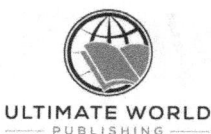

# TESTIMONIALS

~

In this book, *Help Yourself… A Nurse's Guide to Implementing Self-Care*, Lillian teaches self-care in an interesting, fun, and useful way. She offers us suggestions to adapt ways of unhealthy living into healthy living. Every nurse should read this book. It has the potential to prevent burnout and unhealthy stress. It will change the way nurses care for others by promoting self-compassion and wise self-care.

**Niomi Reardon,**
**registered nurse and author of *Stress SOULutions***

Lillian challenges nurses to first prioritize self-care to enable the care of others. She highlights the importance of self-awareness in professional work through her own lived experience. She articulates the domains of life where we can regain control in a way that is thoughtful, helpful, and wise. I commend Lillian for writing and sharing her knowledge, and trust readers will find ways of integrating her advice to the betterment of their own lives.

**Dr Jo Lukins,**
**author of *The Elite: Think Like an Athlete,***
***Succeed Like a Champion***

Wow! Just wow! How I wish this book came out fifteen years ago before I began my career in nursing, or maybe even before I entered nursing school. Lillian illustrated accurately how stress can impact your life in general, particularly for health professionals. When I began my nursing career, I was married, raising two kids, was working in one of the busiest county ERs in Los Angeles and to top that off, I was also working in urgent care as per diem. After a couple of years in the ER, I decided to get my BSN and eventually continued to obtain my MSN specializing in family nurse practitioner. I could not believe the amount of stress I put on my body and as a result, I got really sick.

If this book was around when I entered nursing school, it could've saved me from becoming ill. Nursing is a very stressful job and if you don't learn how to balance out your life as Lillian recommends in this book, potentially, you could end up very sick. I strongly encourage anyone who is thinking about going into nursing, or working as a nurse currently, to pick up this book and implement self-care and apply the recommendations to balance out your life.

**Arwin Kalaw,
certified nurse practitioner**

What an interesting and engaging way to present such crucial and absolutely true methods of dealing with both life and work as a health-care professional. I'm sure I will refer back to these tools repeatedly in the future.

**Sue Whitsell,
certified registered nurse**

Oh wow, your book is beautiful and just what I needed! After a patient told me I had no right to inconvenience her with my vacation when she needed an appointment, I irrationally succumbed and double booked myself to fit her in before I leave! Why did I allow her to control me?! I'm so mad at myself. After reading this book I have realized I am allowing my patients to treat me this way because of hidden fears and our profession's ideal of benevolence which directly relates to our self-worth. We have been taught to give it all away without complaint, but as Lillian points out, this behavior leaves us with nothing left to give. We have defeated our own purpose of "caring for people". Thank you, Lillian. I have learned a cup is neither half full or half empty—it's refillable. Self-care allows us to refill our cup.

**Amy Strocsher,**
**certified family nurse practitioner**

Lilian has been there and done it all in her extensive career as a registered nurse, nurse practitioner and nurse entrepreneur. In her book she shares with us her personal insights on how to holistically take care of ourselves—not only as nurses, but also as women. She has given us a how-to for helping ourselves to overcome our fears, build confidence, and be in control no matter the situation. Regardless if you are a novice or seasoned nurse, this book is a must read.

**Tritia J Murillo,**
**registered nurse and family nurse practitioner**

As a nurse myself, we come from a giving heart and space, and at times we give too much. But what is too much? I question myself all the time as it is so very subjective, and we all have different thresholds. In this book Lillian illustrates ways and methods to look after yourself that are realistic and achievable. As she explains, self-care is a must in our profession, for the mind, body and spirit. This book was a great reminder to myself to not devalue my worth as a nurse and leader, and to remember to fill my cup first, and then share from the overflow. Thank you, Lillian, for sharing your energy and experience with us all.

**MariCruz Bustamante,**
**certified family nurse practitioner**

# CONTENTS

~

Testimonials ..................................................................................iii

Dedication..................................................................................... ix

Introduction................................................................................. xi

Chapter 1: Finding Peace ............................................................. 1

Chapter 2: Complete Control .....................................................13

Chapter 3: Energy Boost ............................................................ 27

Chapter 4: Abundance Now....................................................... 45

Chapter 5: Success Patterns = Rapid Results ........................... 55

Chapter 6: Vision 2 Reality ........................................................ 65

Chapter 7: Ultimate Balance...................................................... 71

Chapter 8: Beyond Guilt .............................................................81

Chapter 9: Unlocking Connection............................................. 89

Chapter 10: Do Your Own Thing............................................... 97

Chapter 11: Heal Yourself ........................................................107

Chapter 12: My Journey with Ayahuasca, Kambo and Bufo ...117

Appendices..................................................................................131

About the Author........................................................................157

Offer 1: Half-Day Self-Care Workshop
    for Health-Care Professionals............................................... 161

Offer 2: Online Self-Care Learning Course
    for Health-Care Professionals...............................................163

Offer 3: Holistic Health Assessment and Coaching.............165

# DEDICATION

~

I would like to dedicate this book to my family, friends, colleagues, and spiritual teachers Mario, Ezequiel and Maria. Thank you for encouraging me to share my stories and allowing me into your lives. I have learned so much from each one of you and am blessed to have such wonderful loving caring people in my life. A special thanks to my husband, Victor; my three daughters, Lillian, Vanessa, and Priscilla; and my three grandchildren, Omar, Amelia, and Athena for their love and support. You mean the world to me. I could not imagine my world without you.

A very special thank you to my mother, Rebeca, my Aunt Silvia, and my Aunt Mirin. It took a village to raise me and each one of you played a very important role in my upbringing in teaching me resilience and not looking at obstacles, but the opportunities life has to offer—and not seeing challenging events as painful experiences but opportunities for growth.

I would like to personally thank you for picking up this book. As a health-care professional you have dedicated your life to helping others and you make our world a better place to live by showing compassion and love to every single person you touch. You are the true definition of angels walking this earth.

## HELP YOURSELF...

If you allow me, I would love to share with you some self-healing techniques I have learned over my thirty years in health care. My wish for you is that you avoid some of the pitfalls I went through. I share my personal stories that I am sure most of you will relate to. My experience is that as nurses and health-care providers we all want to help people feel better, but unfortunately, we forget about our own needs and suffer from stress, anxiety and burnout.

To truly care for others, we must first care for ourselves.

# INTRODUCTION

~

The purpose of this book is to share the tools I have discovered along my pursuit of self-healing, self-discovery, and, most of all, obtaining and maintaining optimum spiritual, emotional, mental, and physical health. This book is for anyone who is in a position that provides care for someone else, but who in the process, is not taking enough care of him or herself.

For nurses and health-care providers the responsibility of caring for others can often come at the expense of caring for ourselves. In putting our patients first, we may experience a variety of worries and health concerns, which if not handled well, can cause us to become ill. This may include anxiety, burnout, declining health, depression, feelings of guilt, lack of energy, and weight gain caused by emotional eating.

In this book, you will learn simple but effective ways to increase your energy, decrease stress and anxiety, and most importantly, prevent burnout. You'll discover tools to help you deal with the daily pressures of the job and proven techniques that allow you to change your feelings of guilt to feelings of empowerment.

When put into practice, these techniques and tools will transform the way you feel and enhance your ability to care for others—for the betterment of both your personal and professional life.

# CHAPTER 1

# *FINDING PEACE*

~

"Calm mind brings inner strength and self-confidence, so that's very important for good health."

**– Dalai Lama**

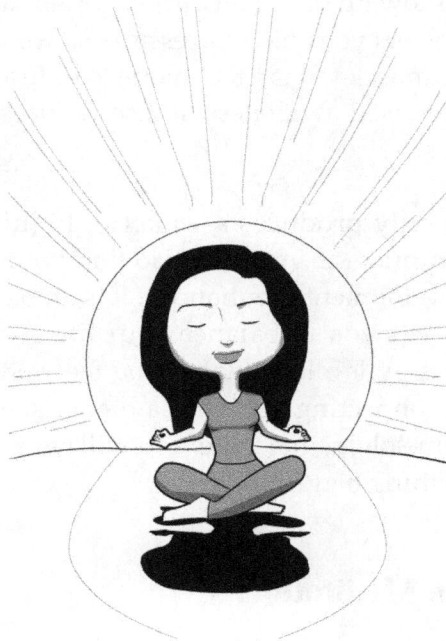

"If we have no peace, it's because we have forgotten that we belong to each other."

**– Mother Teresa**

**D**id you know that meditation increases the gray matter in the brain, and therefore improves our memory and focus? Wow. As nurses, this is incredibly important because we have so many things that we need to remember; not only for our patients and people for whom we care, but also in our personal lives, and for ourselves. For example, if you are a parent, you have a lot to manage and remember when it comes to your everyday routine, including the things that need to get done. And, of course, as we age, our memory does decline.

But, luckily, we can maintain and improve memory through the aid of meditation. Meditation connects us to the source and brings inner peace through the ability of silencing the mind and developing focus toward our main purpose. Meditation slows your heart rate and lowers your blood pressure, slows your breathing, and relaxes your muscles. It is a technique to induce a state of deep relaxation and focused awareness. It also reduces the emotional overload of stress.

Meditation not only produces a wakeful, highly alert mental state, but once in practice, you will also find your inner strength and personal development is enhanced. It is an old and profound method that assists you to balance your life and improve and increase your energy levels. It makes you feel better by reducing your stress and connecting you with a higher source so you can become a problem-solving machine. You will gain a sense that you are part of something bigger.

## Everyone Can Meditate

There are many different types of meditation which makes it possible for everyone to find a practice they can relate to. If you make the effort to meditate every day, your stress levels will decrease, and you will establish a connection while receiving guidance that you perhaps never knew you had within you. When meditation is part of your daily life, you can improve your mind, and your physical and spiritual body. It has been said that meditation boosts your immune system and reduces the incidence of many common ailments including stress, anxiety, high blood pressure, headaches, migraines, digestive disorders, depression, insomnia, long-term pain, and addictions.

There are many people who frown upon meditation. These same people believe it's something to do after eating a bowl of quinoa for lunch and swear it's only done by "hippies." Sadly, they are missing out on a lot of benefits and, with that closed mindset, will likely continue to live life on autopilot, doing the same things over and over, reacting versus responding to situations in their lives. A life that feels as if it is lacking in purpose can ultimately result in levels of depression. With depression comes an increase in stress and the poor memory that we touched on earlier.

Being in that type of mental state may cause you to feel like you are ungrounded and disconnected. It can also cause oversensitivity and a sense of vulnerability in daily situations affecting you at work and home. The ability to be grounded can often lead to making wiser decisions, feeling more focused, and being more present with those around you.

Realistically, meditation is about connecting to the source and finding inner peace through developing the ability to calm the mind and shift your focus toward your true purpose. By incorporating meditation into your daily life, you will experience less physical and mental stress. You will also experience less illness.

You know people can say, "I just cannot meditate. I don't know how other people can do it." The reality is, anyone can meditate. Meditation can be easy and doesn't have to be you sitting down on the floor, legs crossed, eyes closed, with absolute perfect posture. There is a stigma around meditation, frequently heard, that only spiritually inclined people can do it. The reality is that with some simple guidelines and willingness to try, meditation is within the reach of everyone.

# The Many Ways to Meditate

There are many types of meditations. Of course, there is the traditional method of sitting mentioned above, but there are also other ways to meditate that are quite active, including walking and exercising. There are forms of meditation where you ground yourself. There are visual meditations where you can be staring out into the sea or at the sunset. There are auditory forms where you are guided through the meditation by a soothing voice in terms of what to do and how to control your breathing at an even pace, which can make it so much easier to focus. There is transcendental meditation (also known as TM meditation), a simplified seven-step approach to learning how to meditate. There is also Vipassana mindful meditation that teaches you how to be mindful of the here and now using breath control.

Meditation aids were invented to make the whole experience more fulfilling. Some of the tools you can use are crystals, colors, voice-guided music, and creating a space where you will enjoy this path. Using these tools and focusing on the meditation process is truly about giving back to yourself and filling up your own tank so you can do your best for others for whom you are caring for.

Colors that are present in meditation each have their own meanings as described below:

- **Red** promotes leadership, courage, energy, confidence, willpower, and/or initiative. It increases our adrenaline. It's good for people who are experiencing depression, shyness, fear, or fatigue.

- **Orange** promotes and simulates self-esteem, inner strength, creativity, happiness, and/or new ideas. It is also good for people who are experiencing depression, trauma, stress, anxiety, or who want to improve mental clarity.

- **Yellow** promotes cleansing, self-confidence, self-control, mental stimulation, and enhances memory. It is good for people who often experience depression, fatigue, sensitivity to criticism, or lack confidence.

- **Green** promotes balance, personal development, compassion for self, and self-renewal. Green is considered good for people who experience stress, anxiety, self-pity, depression, mood swings, and indecision.

- **Blue** promotes calm, peace, relaxation, slowing down, reduces blood pressure, and can also cool a fever. It is a great color for people who experience insomnia, stress, anxiety, and anger, as well as those who are looking to improve their mental relaxation and patience.

- **Indigo** promotes wisdom, intuition, peace, calm, and inspiration. Indigo is good for people who experience anger, insomnia, anxiety, fear, or repression.

- **Violet** promotes inspiration, imagination, empathy, and self-respect. It can help those who experience stress, anxiety, a lack of confidence, or depression.

- **Pink** promotes calm, affection, compassion, and is good for difficult relationships, anger, aggression, and depression. Pink is also ideal for cleansing.

- **White** is the purest of colors. It is a cleansing color associated with higher ideals. White raises and promotes enthusiasm, wisdom, and healing. White is also good for depression, anxiety, and stress.

- **Black** is the most powerful color because it absorbs the energy. It is best to avoid it if you're experiencing depression.

# Regular Effort and Practice is Key

While discussing meditation, I'd like to share my personal experience of the first time I tried it. I'd read so many books on meditation and attended so many retreats and seminars. After doing much research and reading countless pages, it came down to understanding that with meditation, there is no such thing as a right way or a wrong way to practice it.

What I came to discover was that guided meditation works best for me. Allow me to share my first experience with you. If I am being completely honest, my first experience with meditation was very funny and not at all of what an ideal meditation session should look like. And I am sure some of you may relate and have your own funny day-one meditation stories too.

One day, I chose to set up my meditation space in my bedroom. I shut the door, burned some incense, took off my shoes, and sat on my bed. I took a deep breath, closed my eyes, and pictured a white wall. Now, I didn't choose to imagine a giant blank wall, it was what I was instructed to do to clear my mind from all thoughts. As determined as I was to make this meditation thing work, and however hard I tried to picture this wall, it only lasted about a second. I started to picture my to do list on that white wall and started to stress about everything that needed to get done.

You see, I have a type A-plus personality and always have a list with check points, timelines, and due dates. While focusing on my list, I could also hear the television blasting in the living room and my daughters having an ongoing discussion talking louder than the television. And instead of focusing on this compelling white wall, I quickly became engaged in their conversation. In my mind, I was solving their problems. I came back to my to-do list and got very irritated and upset because I was falling behind with the things I needed to do. This was very stressful. I did not find myself relaxed or calm at all. If anything, I was even more stressed out then when I started the whole process.

There really is no right and wrong in terms of how to meditate. And sometimes our monkey brain is there in the beginning and it may come in and out during our meditation. Monkey brain is a term used in meditation circles when our mind bounces from one idea to another resulting in anxiety and stress.

For the record, every single meditation you participate in will always be different. No two meditation sessions will be the same and not every experience can be as fulfilling as the one before. The important thing is that we keep doing it and we keep on working with it. Refining and improving our meditation practices and getting to a state that ultimately is the best state for ourselves.

## Staying Grounded

There is one meditation that I discovered as a nurse that really made a difference in my life. And that is what we call the grounding meditation. It is a process of bringing yourself fully into your body and connecting with the natural world, (Pachamama) mother earth. It is all about getting outside and finding a patch of grass or finding a tree that you can stand near with your bare feet. Grounding meditation is extremely helpful for us as nurses because we encounter a lot of people in our lives.

We become magnets and make everyone feel good by absorbing all the emotions and stresses from other people and bringing it into our own bodies. At the end of the day, we are tired and drained, which causes us to become extremely unfocused and exhausted. When you practice grounding meditation, you release that unwanted and heavy energy to mother earth, which allows you to feel more relaxed and have a cleared mind that is rid of the negative energy.

Before I begin any meditation, I like to say the following passage: "In this meditation and throughout my life, I invite my guardian angels and spirit guides of the highest light to be with me. All others are not invited and are not to be part of my life or in my life and are not to be present in this meditation."

If you prefer to hold a crystal during meditation, black tourmaline is a wonderful stone for grounding and protecting energies and the aura. You may also use a smoky quartz, which is known to improve connection to the physical world.

The way I like to practice grounding meditation is by going to the park, taking off my shoes and socks, and leaning up against a tree. I put my feet directly on the grass or the soil. Then, I visualize golden rays coming to me and running down my body with my feet firmly on the ground. I also picture roots coming out of my feet and going into the ground, penetrating deep in the soil. The golden light that comes from heaven fills me with unconditional love, knowing I am a nurse and a nurturer, it replenishes my battery.

My mind becomes clear, allowing me to make clearer decisions. As I breathe in, I breathe in unconditional love. As I breathe out, I release all my unwanted emotions and fears. I spend fifteen to thirty minutes practicing grounding meditation. I then give thanks to God and my guides of the highest light for this beautiful blessing and cleansing.

As nurses, we give so much to others. And we are absorbing a lot of their emotions and stresses, some in lower vibrational states. We need to increase our vibrational states so that we can give back a higher vibration to our patients. I refer to higher vibration as clearing away any lower frequency energy you might be carrying. Lower vibrational states can cause decreased energy, poor concentration and a lack of initiative.

I want to share an experience I had with plant medicine. A little over a year ago, my husband and I traveled to Mexico with a group of shamans. I had the opportunity to meditate using plant medicine. It was a life-changing experience for me. I really connected to the universal God, the light source. I got a clearer picture of my purpose in this life. I was given messages about this book and a healing center combining Western and Eastern practices.

My universal God is good, and I accept all good things coming. I was shown a map and in that map was an image of where I should be and where I was at present. I had deviated from my true dharma, my true path. I have spent a large time of my life trying to help others both professionally and personally and, in the process, I had totally forgotten about me. I am sure, as nurses, you can relate to this.

## Learning to Let Go

Thankfully, I have been blessed with having wonderful mentors in my life. My Aunt Mirin told me, "It is not up to you to fix them they are walking their path and you are walking yours. Stop investing time and energy where you don't need to, and you will see how easy your life will be." She said, "That's how we grow; if we don't go through the life challenges that allow us to grow then we will be stagnant. Don't take that experience away from them. You will limit them from growing as individuals."

I felt like someone threw a glass of cold water in my face. I never thought of it that way. Let me tell you that as soon as my mentality changed, the guilt that goes along with not helping enough or not being available 24/7 was completely gone. I started investing that time and energy on improving myself and it's been an awesome experience. Try it and see how your life will change. You will stop attracting chaos in your life because you will no longer be looking for it. Instead, you will be looking for things that bring you peace and happiness.

Meditation with the assistance of plant medicine, or without, can open those channels to connect with a divine source. I was blessed to go to India with my Aunt Mirin and attend the 33rd Kalachakra Initiation where we prayed for everyone in the world. The Dalai Lama said he wakes up every morning at three o'clock in the morning to meditate. There is something special between three o'clock and five o'clock in the morning that connects us to a higher source and a higher self during meditation, allowing us to receive mental clarity and messages.

You may ask yourself, "What if I don't have time to meditate?" As you know, nurses work such long hours. The good news is, meditation can be done at any time. The best place to start on a busy schedule is as you are going to sleep, or during your shower. There is no time limit or place. Your intention just has to be there. YouTube has a one-minute meditation that you can look up if you would like a more visual example.

When something is important to us, we will make time for it. I am a big believer that being comes with the doing. So, let's get you out there and doing some of these meditations. (As a disclosure, do not meditate while driving or operating heavy machinery and check with your doctor before starting meditation practice.)

## Your three action steps
## for this chapter:

1. I want you to go outside and perform your very first grounding meditation and see how you feel. Maybe journal how you feel. Do it for a few days in a row and see how it changes you. The first one might not be mind-blowing, but you never know what the next one will be like. You never know, so just keep doing them.

2. During the next meditation, give your subconscious mind a problem that you've had for a while and would like to see if you can solve over the next few meditations. You might not come up with anything immediately. You might come up with it in a month or so after you have focused on it. Remember solutions can come during meditation and during sleep and dreams, where a person might come and talk to you and give you an idea.

3. Research meditation aids to guide you through your meditations and create a space where you can do meditate on a regular basis.

When you are ready to take the next steps, head to the Appendices at the end of the book for more exercises that will help you make meditation part of your daily life.

# CHAPTER 2

# COMPLETE CONTROL
## DEALING WITH STRESS
## AT WORK AND HOME

"When you undervalue what you do, the world will undervalue who you are."

– Oprah Winfrey

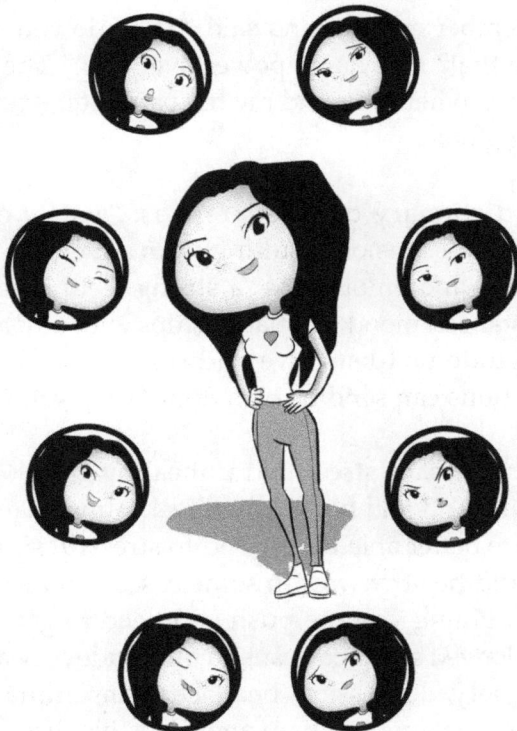

"Self-esteem comes from being able to define the world in your own terms and refusing to abide by the judgments of others."

**– Oprah Winfrey**

When I was a new grad, I worked with a very irrational doctor. He was always very angry and extremely impatient. We worked in the high acuity unit. This doctor used to make me cry every night. He had this terrible attitude toward nurses, like we were beneath him. Yet he came to the senior nurses for help all the time as they were the true experts in the unit. He would arrive at the unit and belittle all the nurses, including me. I remember one night I started crying before I even left my house and my husband said, "What's wrong?" I told him how much I hated going to work, not because of my patients, but because I had to deal with this doctor. I remember my husband said, "Why do you allow him to treat you like that? He has no power over you." The stress I was feeling was overwhelming and my husband's question struck me like a lightning bolt.

The Oxford dictionary defines stress as: "a state of mental or emotional strain or tension resulting from adverse or demanding circumstances," and emotion as "a strong feeling deriving from one's circumstances, mood, or relationships with others." Emotions function to guide us to survive and thrive—but holding on to negative emotions can send us on a downward spiral.

Reducing unnecessary stress and unhealthy emotions takes the strain off your mind and body. You'll feel calmer, can think more clearly, and are better able to respond to stressful situations in an appropriate and healthy way. In some cases, a little stress can be motivating in giving you the push you need to get things done. However, prolonged stress can cause a multitude of health concerns including anxiety, depression, headaches, insomnia, high blood pressure, muscle pain, back pain and digestive disorders.

COMPLETE CONTROL

## Cultivating a Healthy Mindset

By removing anxiety and unnecessary stress, you release unwanted and unneeded emotions and thoughts that block your paths to success. Uncontrolled stress and emotions can make us physically and mentally ill. It affects your mood and decision-making process. You become unaware, out of control, and operate on autopilot, reacting to situations instead of responding to them. Harboring negative feelings, such as envy, resentment, and fear have been linked to inflammation and a higher risk of disease. When you can switch your focus to positive feelings such as abundance and happiness, you'll not only enjoy an enhanced sense of well-being, you'll also lower your risk of disease and inflammation.

As a result of uncontrolled stress and negative emotions, we can experience irrational thinking. A decision can be made in a split second, and if you are angry or disappointed, you are not making sound decisions. It is best to take a step back, take a deep breath, and maybe write down the pros and cons. Think about it, analyze it and then make your decision. We, as nurses, are responsible for the welfare of those in our care. Our patients and their family members rely on us to always maintain a sound decision-making process.

Some of the tools that can be used to assist us in releasing negative emotions and stress include acupressure, tai chi, yoga, massage, reflexology, counseling, emotional freedom techniques (EFT), and transformation therapy. I went to see an amazing transformational coach at the Radical Aliveness Institute in Los Angeles. She is passionate about helping people overcome their fears and build self-confidence. She really helped me with my own transformation and taught me how to take my power back and be true to myself.

Back when I was working in the high acuity unit, my husband's question regarding my work situation gave me new clarity. I became determined to go to work with a calmer mindset so I could be ready to make better decisions for me and my patients. Well, that night I wiped my tears and put on my big girl pants and drove to work, and like clockwork this particular doctor came in yelling and screaming. One of my patients needed an amiodarone IV push and our protocol stated we must have a nurse, a respiratory tech, a physician, and a crash cart by the patient's bedside before it was performed. When he came to my patient's room he stated, "I need amiodarone IV push now!" I said, "I need to call the respiratory tech and I need to get the crash cart." He repeated, "Now!"

That was the day I stood up for myself and I called the charge nurse, explained the situation and guess who got in big trouble? In this case, irrational thinking might have caused improper care to the patient, but we as nurses must remain calm and collected. We are the voice for our patients, and they trust we will take care of them. The doctor came back the following days much quieter. I share my story because if you are working in an environment that is not healthy or one where you do not feel appreciated or acknowledged as part of a team, it is very important that you do not allow yourself to fall into that negativity. It is important that you do not harbor unhealthy emotions that may lead you to illness in the future.

I have four key guidelines that I follow to ensure my thoughts and emotions are healthy, to allow me to provide the best care for my colleagues and patients:

1. Work on yourself and learn how to acknowledge the emotions you are feeling and not suppress them, because they will come back to haunt you.

2. Be true to yourself always.

3. Stand up for yourself.

4. Remain cool and collected.

In contrast to my earlier story, I have since been blessed to work for some exceptional companies that have weekly meetings with the providers, care managers, nurses, office staff, managers, and even the owners are present. They are constantly looking to improve the work environment for everyone. I can honestly say, aside from having a happy staff, the patients also benefit because when there is collaboration in care and good communication the flow of care runs so much better and the outcomes are wonderful.

Don't be disappointed if you don't work in a nurturing environment and give up hope. They are out there you just have to be proactive and seek them out. They really do exist.

## Stress and Your Health

You might ask yourself can stress and uncontrolled emotions affect my health? The answer is YES. Being in the health care field for thirty years now, I have seen this firsthand. While studying natural medicine, I completed a course in Chinese medicine, including herbology. I learned that in Chinese medicine it is believed that each organ can be affected by emotions which can block the Qi, the vital force, or energy force, that animates the body internally. For example:

- anxiety may affect our lungs and our large intestine

- frustration, anger, resentment, or irritability, may cause high blood pressure and headaches, and may affect our liver and gallbladder

- happiness and joy may affect our heart and small intestine

- grief, sadness, or depression may affect our lungs and large intestine

- fear, insecurity, and indecisiveness may affect our kidneys, adrenals, and bladder

- worry, obsessive thinking, and nervousness may affect our spleen and stomach

I've also learned negative emotions can impact our immune system, reducing natural killer cell activity and antibody production, causing increased susceptibility to colds and other viral infections.

## Natural Remedies That Assist with Emotions

There are many natural remedies available that can help to alleviate negative emotions and bring you back to a calmer state of mind. The following are some that I have tried and found to be effective.

Flower remedies that can help you overcome a negative state of mind:

- Agrimony: hiding worries behind a brave face, concealing problems
- Centaury: weak-willed, exploited or imposed upon, anxious to please
- Elm: overwhelmed by responsibility
- Hornbeam: procrastination
- Larch: lack of self-confidence, feelings of inferiority, fear of failure
- Pine: guilty feelings and self-reproachful

Essential oils that can alleviate ailments:

- Anxiety: chamomile and lavender
- Insomnia: chamomile and lavender
- Headaches: peppermint and eucalyptus

Gemstones that assist with emotions:

- Citrine: increase energy and self-esteem, enhances creativity, and brings inner calm
- Lapis lazuli: promotes self-worth, integrity, and wisdom
- Moonstone: strengthens intuition, aids in dieting, and alleviates stress
- Pyrite: increases energy, focus, and confidence
- Turquoise: used for courage, success, and personal power

A simple technique used to relieve stress headaches:

- Pinch the web between your thumb and forefinger with the thumb and forefinger of our other hand. Squeeze for one to two minutes, repeat three to four times, then switch hands and repeat. This takes very little time and is very effective.

## How You Can Reduce Stress Today

The combination of high-pressure work and the hectic pace of life means that many health-care professionals (and much of the general population) are experiencing ongoing stress. By introducing some simple daily techniques and healthy habits, you can significantly lower your stress levels in both the short and longer term. Here are five things you can do today to reduce stress in your life.

1. **Rest.** Most of us were taught this in nursing school, but, for whatever reason, most nurses I know seem to feel rest does not pertain to them. Trust me. I went through that phase, too, and it's guaranteed to cause nurse burnout if not addressed. It is very important to get plenty of sleep. One of the things I do is look at my schedule, and if I start work at seven o'clock in the morning, that means I must get up at 5:30am. I count back seven to eight hours. This

means I go to bed no later than 9:30pm. I set my bedtime alarm for nine o'clock at night when I'll start getting ready for bed.

I recommend putting your phone or any electric devices away from you to keep you from being distracted. You can set your alarm thirty minutes prior to bedtime. This will give you time to meditate, pray, and practice deep breathing exercises before settling in for the night. During my prayer and meditation, I practice gratitude. I always start with thanking God for my children, grandchildren, husband and spiritual teachers. Then I extend it to my parents, siblings, cousins, friends, and colleagues. If I have anything that is weighing me down, I ask God and my spirit guides of the highest light to enlighten me and to help me with my concern or problem. I find this is very effective in giving me a restful sleep and for reminding me I am not alone in this journey we call life.

2.  **Laughter.** God knows that, as nurses, we have an uncanny sense of humor. This is a humor that only nurses and people in the health care industry can appreciate. We can talk and laugh about some pretty grotesque events—all while eating at the family table—and our family and friends are looking at us like "what is wrong with you." I think God gave us that gift because he knew it would come in handy in releasing work stress.

    Laughter is so important for relaxing and letting loose. Do things you enjoy and laugh, laugh, laugh. I have been very fortunate in having people around me who make me laugh and let loose. As I stated earlier, I am a type A-plus personality and can be very rigid at times. I am grateful for the people around me—my husband, children and grandchildren—who remind me to let loose, laugh, and not be so uptight.

Laughing promotes your thymus gland to produce T cells (your killer cells), which play a very important role in keeping you healthy. Laughter has been known to aid in the healing process. Levels of cortisol and epinephrine decrease after laughter, reversing the stress-induced inflammatory cascade. Sometimes I will go to a theme park and get on a roller coaster and pray to God that I don't fall out and die. Then I laugh, laugh, laugh. I consider this a two for one. It's a great stress reliever—try it sometime.

3. **Pamper yourself.** I can see most of you reading this and saying, "really, and when exactly is that supposed to happen?" It's like everything else in our lives—pencil it in just as you do all your other activities. If you have small children or are caring for elderly parents, try organizing a few hours to get away and be by yourself. Get a manicure, pedicure, facial, thirty-minute massage, or some energy healing. The key is to make time for yourself.

What do you enjoy? We spend so much time and energy taking care of everyone else that we don't do things we enjoy. Ask yourself if money or time were not an obstacle, what would you love to do. Do you want to travel, go to a spa, get your hair washed and cut, take a day off and go to the beach, the park, or an amusement park? Do you want to try a new activity? What is it that brings joy to your heart?

I enjoy traveling and I know that when I travel, I get more creative. I enjoy talking to people from different countries and states and learning from them. I see the world and people through a different lens. I feel like I get more assertive and start putting some of my needs first. This is a good thing. I take more risks and get out of what I call, "the hamster wheel." I challenge myself and, even though I am afraid, I do it because I know that is how I will continue to grow. If traveling is not for you, maybe joining a network, learning something new, taking some classes or self-improvement courses will work. We only live this life once, so it's good to push the envelope and try new things, meet new people, see new places, challenge yourself, and allow yourself to grow. Don't get caught up in the hamster wheel.

4. **Be Assertive.** Nurses are the most resilient people I know. But, for whatever reason when we are new grads, we forget this, and we get intimidated easily and some of us get pushed around. I know, as a new grad, I did for a bit until I woke up. If you are a new grad or you are new to a position, I am speaking to you. Give yourself credit that you made it this far because you have what it takes. Never doubt yourself and please don't allow others to instill their fears in you. When I encounter people like that, I remember it's not about me; they are dealing with their own insecurities.

One of the most life-changing experiences I had was when I was forty-six. I had a great job in California with wonderful benefits. I worked with great colleagues, had good friends, and made decent money for a nurse practitioner. Even though this was a secure job, I felt like I was not living my dharma. I felt hollow on the inside. I kept on remembering the map I saw in my meditation and I knew staying in California was only going to push me further away from my path. So, I quit my job and decided to move back to Arizona, but to a different city than where I previously lived. I had no job and I had no home. But deep inside I knew it was the right move for me. My family and friends all thought I was crazy, and they asked me, "Are you okay? Where will you live? Where will you work?" My answer at the time was, "I'm not sure."

Long story short, I found a great job and a beautiful home in Arizona. In the beginning it was very difficult, and I cried because my new job was so different. It really pushed me out of my comfort zone, and it was very challenging. I felt like I was not prepared for it. You see, I was spoiled in my previous job. This new job took some adjustment and time. I remember one day after work I was crying in my room and my husband asked, "What's wrong?" And, I said, "I don't know how I can help my patients? I don't know if I am the right person or if I am even in the right place. I think I should have stayed in California where everything was easier." He asked me, "What chapter are you working on now?" I was currently writing this book. I said in a very angry voice, "What does that have to do with anything? You're not listening to me. I'm telling you I don't think I'm qualified for this job. I think I made a big mistake in leaving." And, he asked me again, "What chapter are you working on?" I answered, *"How to Handle Your Emotions. Why?"* And he just looked at me and then I laughed, and he laughed, and I said, "Oh my God, you are right. I was stuck on what to write about, but now I know."

Then the words just flowed through me and, oddly enough, my job got easier and after that the block was lifted both at work and with my writing. The reason I share this story is because when we are going through difficult times in our lives, it is very important to ask, "What is the lesson I need to learn now?" It is okay to take risks and grow. It's not always easy in the beginning, but as nurses we are natural chameleons and can adapt to any situation. I encourage you to take risks, to challenge yourself. You will grow both personally and professionally.

5.  **Simplify.** Where to begin? This is big for me because I think something is wrong when things are too simple and there is no stress. I have been dealing with codependency my whole life, as many of us as nurses and health-care providers are. I want to take it on and help everyone. I

can fix any situation and take away other people's pain, suffering, and problems. I had to learn that some things just have to be left alone. As my Aunt Mirin taught me, if I don't, I am taking away that person's opportunity to learn. I am hurting, not helping. I just need to step back and allow the process to happen.

Once I did this, my life became less complicated, less stressful. I really have to practice this and constantly remind myself. We should simplify our lives as much as we can. I stopped taking on too much and stopped overextending myself. I used to volunteer for everything and stretched myself so thin I was always walking around angry, impatient, and upset, the total opposite of what I wanted to do, which was to help. Not anymore. I value myself and my time. If I can help, I will. If I cannot, I'm okay with saying, "I'm sorry, I cannot right now. Maybe another time."

One of the lessons I learned in my new job in Arizona is that it's okay to accept help. It's okay to delegate. When we don't accept help, we also take away the blessing from the person who wanted to help us. This is a new concept for me, as I was brought up in a family where you don't ask for help under any circumstance. You made your bed; you sleep in it. This has taken so much stress away from me. I thank God every day for allowing me to have the courage to leave my comfort zone and try something new. I feel like I am living my dharma and I am giving back. I am back on track, full speed ahead.

I have learned that our emotions really do affect our decision process. When our emotions are activated, they are done so to illicit one of the survival behaviors. That is why it is so important, as nurses, that we are constantly evaluating our emotions. We work with so many people and so many different personalities that this can become a juggling act. We must remember, we are there to help and cannot allow environmental or even personal circumstances to get in the way.

When I studied holistic wellness, I was taught: "When a feeling arises in reaction to a situation, become aware of the true feeling and acknowledge it."

We learned that uncontrolled emotions can cause depression, anxiety, and lead to smoking, drinking, illegal drug use, overeating, insomnia, etc. So, let's try everything in our power not to allow emotions to make us ill.

# Your three action steps
# for this chapter:

1.  What are some of the things you can incorporate in your daily routine today to decrease stress and negative emotions in your life?

2.  List some of the physical and mental symptoms caused by uncontrolled emotions and uncontrolled stress.

3.  Write down some techniques you can use to control negative emotions, such as praying, meditating, exercise, etc.

When you are ready to take the next steps, head to the Appendices at the end of the book for more exercises that will help you manage stress effectively.

# CHAPTER 3

# ENERGY BOOST

~

"The doctor of the future will no longer treat the human frame with drugs but rather will cure and prevent disease with nutrition."

– **Thomas Edison**

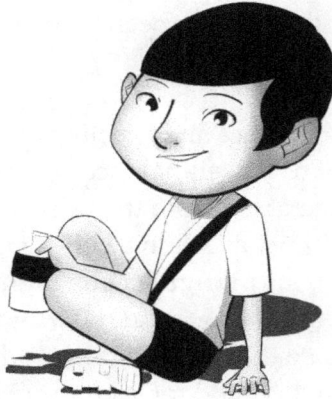

"Our food should be our medicine and our medicine should be our food."

– **Hippocrates**

**A**s nurses we are so used to turning to our medical system to heal our patients. This means we sometimes forget that our own health begins with the "medicines" found in our gardens and kitchens. Did you know people who exercise, eat well, meditate, pray, practice gratitude, and feel loved and cared for, tend to report better mental and physical health than those who don't?

Have you ever wished you could better regulate your mood and mind? A well-balanced diet that includes poultry, fatty fish, cruciferous vegetables, and B vitamins can help maintain a harmonious balance and improve your mood. A diet high in refined sugars and processed foods has been known to cause forgetful, foggy mind, and inflammation in the body. It can increase fatigue and lower your energy levels. Some people also experience depression and melancholy. An unhealthy diet depletes the body's reserve and can lead to illness and disease. It can cause mood swings, weight gain, and obesity. Sugar, caffeinated beverages, alcohol, and high-fat foods have also been known to cause hormonal imbalances.

Are you seeking greater balance and a feeling of equilibrium? Start by focusing on your food. A well-balanced diet should contain a variety of fruits and vegetables, from the full-color spectrum such as berries, eggplant, plums, avocados, bell peppers, cucumbers, nopal (Mexican cactus), and arugula. The pigment in the fruits and vegetables contain natural antioxidants which your body uses to balance free radicals, so they don't damage other cells. Eating a healthy and balanced diet is good for your mind and body—you'll enjoy increased mental clarity, higher energy levels, and improved mental and physical health.

Looking for a happiness boost? Foods such as eggs, salmon, nuts, and seeds can increase serotonin levels. Serotonin is your happy hormone. Serotonin in the brain is thought to regulate anxiety, happiness, and mood. Low levels of serotonin have been associated with depression.

The Mediterranean diet is considered one of the healthiest approaches to eating. It is big on fresh foods and healthy fats such as fruits, vegetables, whole grains, beans, legumes, olive oil, and nuts. Fish, cheese, yogurt, poultry, and eggs are eaten moderately, and red meat only occasionally. This style of eating encourages you to limit processed foods and refined sugars. I always advise my patients that if it comes in a box or you have to drive by the box to order your meal, it generally is not very healthy for you.

Some of the unhealthiest foods are cereal, sugary coffee drinks, soda pop, processed food, white bread, white sugar, white flour, white rice, processed meats, fried foods, and alcohol. If your current diet consists mainly of these, introducing more fresh foods into your daily meals will be highly beneficial for your health.

## What About Detoxification?

Detoxification is a way to cleanse our bodies and rid them of toxins and debris that we have accumulated over the years. It cleans out our blood and gives us mental clarity. It's also a great time to practice meditation and prayer. The way I explain it to my patients is, it's like when you change the oil filter in your car. You don't continue running your car without having regular tune-ups. Our liver is our filter and it needs a break. Remember, the emotions that can affect our liver include anger, frustration, resentment, irritability, rage, bitterness, and disappointment.

One of your liver's jobs is to remove waste products and toxins from your body. It is also responsible for filtering the blood coming from the digestive tract before passing it to the rest of the body. The liver detoxifies chemicals and metabolizes drugs. As it does so, it secretes bile that ends up back in the intestine. What does a proper detoxification do? It allows your organs to rest properly. It improves circulation. It refuels your body by promoting elimination and stimulating your liver, allowing more oxygen to the organs and your brain.

How do you know if you need a detox? Are you experiencing mental fog, digestive issues, bloating, cramping, constipation, fatigue, aches, pains, bad breath, or insomnia? If you answered yes to some of the questions above, a detox might benefit you. Even acne, allergies, itchy skin, rashes, congestion, memory fog, poor concentration, and ear pressure or ringing in the ears could be a sign that your kidney, liver or colon could do with a detox.

Always consult your health-care provider before you start a detox. When I detox, I make sure I take extra naps. I drink plenty of water, practice deep breathing exercises, dry brush my skin, walk, and, most importantly, pray, and meditate.

I personally use the Flor-Essence 7-Day Purification Program at least twice a year. You can purchase this at most health food stores or on Amazon and you just follow the directions on the box. I would encourage you to start it on a day off as chances are you will be using the restroom more frequently than usual. The second detox I practice is getting one gallon of distilled water and adding twenty teaspoons of lemon juice, organic lemons, twenty teaspoons grade A maple syrup, and two teaspoons of cayenne pepper. Mix this and drink it throughout the day. This fast can be done from twenty-four hours up to ten days. I would start with twenty-four hours. This is also recommended on your day off.

When you stop the fast, eat fruits in the morning for breakfast and vegetables for lunch and dinner, limiting protein to fish and chicken, avoiding red meat and pork as much as possible.

So, what will you experience when you detox? Some of you will feel fatigued. Go ahead and sleep, get some rest. This is when your body restores itself. Some of you will have headaches. This is expected, especially if you're coming off caffeine and sugary foods. Make sure you're drinking plenty of water and getting plenty of rest. Practice your deep breathing exercises. While fasting, take walks as this helps in the elimination of toxins. But, avoid strenuous exercise during the fast.

In addition to a full detox, I also drink the following green drink two to three times a week.

**Ingredients:**

- handful of spinach
- one or two celery stalks
- one handful of broccoli flower
- one handful of kale
- two slices of turmeric root
- one small cucumber
- one handful of parsley
- juice of one lemon
- two slices of ginger root
- a glass of water

**Method:** Blend it altogether and drink in the morning or at lunch.

The rest of the days I substitute a meal with the following protein shake.

**Ingredients:**

- one scoop vegan protein shake
- one scoop brewer's yeast
- one teaspoon matcha green tea powder
- a tablespoon of MCT oil
- a glass of water

**Method:** Blend it all together and drink in place of a meal. I drink this shake to substitute for breakfast or lunch, not dinner because of the green tea. It will boost your energy and will cause insomnia.

# Healthy Body and Mind Essentials

As nurses, it is essential to get some daily exercise. The recommendation is thirty to forty-five minutes, five to seven days per week, to the point where you perspire. If you are over forty years of age, be sure to include some weight lifting, because we lose muscle as we get older. Try five or ten-pound weights, resistant bands, or use your own body weight in exercises such as push-ups, pull-ups, sit-ups and planks. However, before you start an exercise program, be sure to check with your health-care provider.

It's also important to include relaxation techniques in your daily life. We are awesome at teaching our patients how to practice them, but we often forget about ourselves. You can choose whichever form appeals to you, whether it is prayer, meditation, yoga, practicing daily gratitude, or all the above. Regular relaxation practice will help you feel better and get a good night's sleep.

I also include spiritual awareness and forgiveness in my daily routine. This is another thing that is quite difficult for me. I tend to harbor ill emotions, but during my experience with plant medicine, I discovered I can bring illness to myself by not forgiving circumstances or situations that have hurt me in the past. Forgive and let go of resentment—not for them, but for you.

Another common theme amongst nurses is that many of us battle with weight issues. One of the big reasons for this is because of the emotions we harbor, it's easy to fall into the trap of emotional eating. I have been guilty of this in the past.

Now, when I am faced with eating without purpose, I ask myself a couple of questions:

- Am I having any feelings of insecurity, vulnerability, fear, or loss of control of circumstances and situations around me?
- Am I tired, sleepy, or overextending myself?

If the answer is yes, then I take a couple of deep breaths and pray about it, or journal about it. I might even walk away from the meal for a bit to see if I really am hungry or if I am stress eating again. I am really committed to making a conscious effort to stop eating without purpose.

My Aunt Silvia, may she rest in peace, taught me that your body is your temple, so treat it as that and don't abuse it. Cherish it, love all of it and don't deprive it. This is still a work in progress for me, but I am doing better as I now take time to acknowledge what I feel as opposed to just eating breakfast, lunch, and dinner in one sitting.

## How Supplements Can Help

Because our land is not as rich in minerals as it once was, I take supplements. When I studied alternative medicine, I learned the importance of supplementing with vitamins, minerals, herbs and homeopathic remedies. I would like to share some of what I discovered with you. Please feel free to continue your own research on them and see which ones might benefit you.

## Supplements to lower stress and support the adrenal gland:

Your adrenal glands are located at the top of each kidney. Two adrenal hormones produced by the adrenal glands are cortisol and aldosterone. Too much stress may cause elevated hormones resulting in anxiety, depression, digestive problems, weight gain, and memory impairment. The following supplements can help:

- **B complex vitamins** boost energy levels and help maintain normal levels of adrenal structure and function

- **Vitamin C with bioflavonoids** is an antioxidant and helps with the production of cortisol and helps us maintain a healthy immune system

- **Ginseng** supports the adrenal glands to increase stamina and reduce lethargy

- **Ashwagandha** acts by regulating cortisol levels. If cortisol is too high, it will lower it. If cortisol is too low, it will raise it. It also has an antioxidant property

- **Holy basil** helps with stress and anxiety, and may increase endurance

- **Maca root** aids cortisol and blood sugar regulation and has a calming effect

- **Probiotics** assist in maintaining a healthy digestive system that allows for better absorption of nutrients and supplements

## Supplements that will help calm your nerves:

- **B complex** are important in keeping the brain and nervous system healthy and maintaining calmness, healthy skin, and muscle tone

- **Vitamin D** increases the body's absorption of calcium, phosphorus, and magnesium which may promote calm nerves resulting in a healthy mood, improved cognitive and cardiovascular function, immune response, and muscle and bone strength

- **Valerian root** calms and sooths the central nervous system and is used for insomnia, nervous tension, anxiety, and stress

## Supplements and oils to reduce insomnia:

- **Chamomile tea** works as a sedative for the nervous system and may also help to decrease anxiety

- **Passionflower tea** helps improve sleep and may help with anxiety

- **Lavender essential oil** is calming and soothing and may be beneficial in reducing stress

- **Tart cherry juice,** (a natural source of melatonin, the sleep producing hormone) improves sleep

## Supplements and foods to improve your liver function:

- **Artichokes** support bile production and are said to have a protective effect on liver cells

- **Milk thistle** inhibits inflammation and stimulates new liver cell production

- **Beets** protect the liver from oxidative stress and chronic inflammation

- **Licorice root** promotes the liver's ability to filter out toxins (but is not recommended if you have high blood pressure)

- **Burdock tea** assists in healing a damaged liver

## Supplements to boost your immune system:

- **Vitamin C with bioflavonoids** is important in energy production and inflammation reduction

- **Selenium** is a powerful antioxidant that has been shown to improve immune system function

- **Mushroom extracts** containing reishi, maitake, and shiitake are a powerful antiviral agent, and immune system modulator

- **Echinacea** aids antiviral and antimicrobial activity and its ability to support the immune system function

- **Zinc** gives the body what it requires to develop and activate T cells which are important players in the immune system

- **Colloidal silver** contains properties that are antiviral, antifungal, and antibacterial

- **Goldenseal** also contains properties that are antiviral, antifungal, and antibacterial

- **Elderberry tea** is rich in flavonoids and is an antioxidant

- **Garlic** contains allicin, a powerful antibiotic

## Supplements for mind and memory:

- **Vitamin C** protects the brain from damage caused by oxidative stress

- **Vitamin E** is an antioxidant, a substance that protects the body from damage caused by free radicals

- **Vitamin D3** promotes healthy mood, cognitive and cardiovascular function, immune response, and muscle and bone strength

- **Omega-3 fatty acids, DHA and EPA** are fundamental to the structure and functioning of all the cell membranes

- **DHA** also supports healthy memory and overall cognition

- **Ginkgo** helps alleviate memory loss and improve concentration by promoting healthy blood flow

## Be Mindful of Your Meals

Feel like you don't have time to plan or pack healthy meals? One method is to pre-pack your meals by cooking several healthy meals on your day off and freezing them. There are many sites on YouTube and Pinterest that can guide you to healthy meal preps.

I also enjoy going to farmers markets where I find good quality fruits and vegetables. Most are reasonably priced and having delicious fresh produce in the pantry and fridge inspires me to make healthy food choices. If you find you often have to eat something on the run or eat out due to a hectic work schedule, where possible choose something that is baked or broiled. Instead of fries, choose a salad; instead of soda or juice, choose water or unsweetened tea. Most takeout places now offer healthier choices. And make sure you always pack a snack that includes fresh fruit and fresh vegetables.

It's very important to monitor your carbohydrate intake and sugar intake. The recommended carbohydrate intake, for women, is thirty to forty-five grams per meal, including snacks. For men, it's forty-five to sixty grams per meal, including snacks. If you are trying to lose weight, it is recommended to eat less carbs. For example, women the recommendation is thirty grams per meal, including snacks, and for males forty-five grams per meal, including snacks. When choosing carbs, try to choose dark green vegetables and low glycemic fruit. Avoid processed food, white bread, white sugar, white flour, and white rice as much as possible.

## Seven Ways to Stay Healthy

You might ask yourself, what steps can I take to stay healthy? Where do I start? Here are seven things you can do today to prevent disease.

1. **Control your emotions.** As discussed in Chapter 2, emotions can cause disease and each emotion affects a certain organ. By practicing biomagnetism, meditation, yoga, breathing techniques, and effective communication, you can release these emotions.

2. **Build your immune system.** It is very important to build your immune system to be strong and healthy. I describe it to my patients in the following way: Imagine you are in a room and you have four strong solid walls, a solid roof, and a solid floor. Then you have a stressor that shows up in your life. If you are not exercising and not eating healthy, you have a weak immune system. If you do not effectively deal with the stressor, one of your walls is knocked down. Now you have an open gateway for bacteria and disease to enter. It can be as simple as a cold or as severe as cancer. Then more stressors come to your life. More walls get knocked down. This makes you more vulnerable to disease.

   Our jobs are extremely stressful. People trust us with their lives and their health, and they trust that we will take care of them. We work with less support staff each day, in many different stressful situations. It is vital that you take care of yourselves and build up your immune system so that you can keep your walls, roof, and floor solid and secure at all times.

3. **Reduce inflammation.** This is super important. Some common triggers include smoking, processed food, coffee, white sugar, white bread, white flour, white rice, preservatives, refined sugars, cakes, pies, cookies, candy, soda, dairy, wheat, and alcohol. This can trigger a leaky gut syndrome, arthritis, pain, headaches, insomnia, and other diseases. To offset this, I take sublingual turmeric herb, a high-quality fish oil supplement, and one tablespoon of apple cider vinegar in four ounces of warm water daily. Just remember to brush your teeth after drinking the apple cider vinegar as it can wear out your enamel. Fasting is another great way to decrease inflammation in the body.

4. **Get plenty of rest.** This is extremely difficult for us as nurses. What is sleep? I'm being sarcastic here. We work eight hours, twelve hours, some of us have even worked sixteen hours. We work day, evening and night shifts. Some of our jobs require us to be on call. Our internal clock is so confused. I know many of my colleagues suffer from insomnia due to a crazy work schedule. To get a good night's sleep, I drink four ounces of tart cherry juice which contains natural melatonin. Drink it thirty minutes before you go to bed and see if it helps. If you don't like the taste, there is an over-the-counter melatonin, however, I prefer the sublingual one. Also, soaking in the tub, meditating, and practicing breathing exercises may help you unwind and obtain proper sleep. I have, in the past, had a habit of taking power naps, to charge my batteries and allow me to finish my shifts.

5. **Maintain a healthy diet.** Include antioxidants and supplements in your daily life. Enjoy foods that are known to be a good source of antioxidant such as pecans, blueberries, strawberries, artichokes, goji berries, raspberries, kale, beets, and spinach. These are only a few, there are many more. Some supplements can also provide you with antioxidants

including beta carotene, lutein, selenium, and vitamin A, C, and E. Again, these are only a few examples. I eat plenty of fruits and vegetables and include fiber and omega-3 fatty acids in my diet.

I also drink a one ounce shot of wheat grass twice a month on a weekend that I am off. If you are going to try this, do it on your day off as it may stimulate your bowels. Wheat grass provides a concentrated amount of nutrients, including iron, calcium, magnesium, amino acid, chlorophyll, and vitamin A, C, and E. It's rich nutrient content boosts immunity, kills harmful bacteria in the digestive system, and rids the body of waste. A diet high in fiber slows down the rate that sugar is absorbed into the bloodstream, while also moving it faster through your intestine, which can help signal that you are full. Fiber cleans your colon, cleaning out bacteria and other buildup in your intestine and reducing your risk for colon cancer. Some foods high in fiber include apples, bananas, oranges, raspberries, mango, dark-colored vegetables, brown rice, beans, and legumes. Supplements used to cleanse and protect the liver include milk thistle, burdock, and green tea.

6. **Get exercise.** Regular exercise is essential to our health in many ways, but one of the lesser known and key benefits is that it moves our lymph system. Unlike our circulatory system, where our heart is a pump, our lymphatic system lacks a pump. So, it is vital we move to stimulate our lymphatic system. One way to explain it is to imagine you take out your garbage on garbage pickup day and the truck doesn't come by to pick it up. The following week, you take out two containers instead of one, and, again, the garbage truck does not come by. The third week you take out three containers of garbage and, again, no one shows up to pick your garbage. This is what happens with your

~ 40 ~

lymphatic system when you don't move. Your lymphatic system becomes clogged, as your lymph functions are unable to clear out the waste. This system plays a key role in your body's defense against illness. Its main job is to move lymph to clear fluids that contain white blood cells that help the body fight infection. If you don't move, you can't clear it. That's why it's important to move. When you move, you keep the flow going and prevent an accumulation of garbage. So, what does your lymphatic system consist of? This is a great question. Your lymphatic system includes your lymph nodes, your lymph ducts, and your lymph vessels.

7. **Detox and fast every four months.** Many people are skeptical of the power of a healthy detox. However, I believe this is the best way you can give your spirit, mind, and body a break. What do I mean by this? Well, if you think about a healthy fast, it will give you mental clarity and improve your digestion. It is also a great time to connect with your inner self and our universal God light source.

We all need to find the right combination of self-care for ourselves. As I have spent many years experimenting with what works best for me, I will summarize my recipe for personal health here:

- I include as many fruits (mostly berries) and vegetables as I can in my diet.

- I take a sublingual B complex with B-12 daily vitamin, a sublingual colloidal silver, selenium and a high-quality omega.

- I walk thirty to forty-five minutes at least five days a week and do my breathing exercises once or twice a day.

- If I have a very stressful day, I watch a comedy show or movie or listen to a comedian and laugh until I cry. There are studies that show that when you laugh, your thymus gland produces T cells. These are your killer cells. We need them to keep us healthy.

- If I don't have time for a full movie, I will soak in the tub. I will add two cups of baking soda, two cups of Epsom salt one handful of Himalayan salt, and listen to some relaxing music. I soak for at least twenty minutes and listen to my affirmations and pray.

While reading this chapter have you considered what small changes you could start to make in your life to improve your health?

~

# Your three action steps
# for this chapter:

1.  Write down three simple steps you can start today to stay healthy.

2.  Choose a couple of supplements that may be of benefit to you and include them in your daily routine.

3.  Find a way to incorporate thirty to forty-five minutes of exercise and movement into your daily routine.

When you are ready to take the next steps, head to the Appendices at the end of the book for more exercises that will help you nourish your body with healthy food.

~

# CHAPTER 4

# ABUNDANCE NOW

"Develop an attitude of gratitude and give thanks for everything that happens to you, knowing that every step forward is a step toward achieving something bigger and better than your current situation."

— **Brian Tracy**

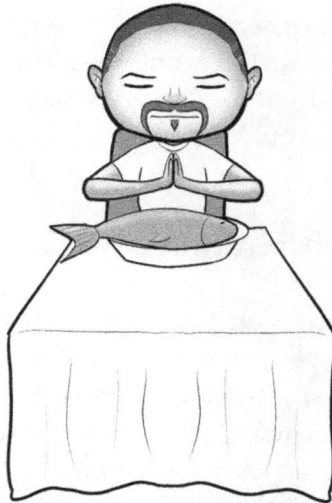

"Gratitude is the healthiest of all human emotions. The more you express gratitude for what you have, the more likely you will have even more to express gratitude for."

— **Zig Ziglar**

really felt stuck in my early twenties and thirties. I was always taught to be grateful for waking up in the morning and being able to live another day, but as I got older, I was in survival mode and I didn't always practice gratitude. I got caught up in life and did not practice what I was taught as a child. When I turned thirty, I was really depressed and felt like I was never going to get ahead. We were under a lot of stress at home. I remember it was late and I was watching infomercials and eating rocky road ice cream, eating my emotions as usual, just feeling sorry for myself.

My husband walked into the living room and said, "What's wrong?" I explained that I've just turned thirty and have not reached any of the goals I have set for myself. This can't possibly be my life. There has to be more to my life. I was stuck, and I was lost.

If I hadn't found a solution, my life would have continued there on that couch. I would have become more miserable, more depressed and my weight gain would have continued. Yet I did find a solution. I became reacquainted with a strategy I had learnt as a child and I want to teach that to you.

## The Power of Daily Gratitude

By incorporating daily gratitude into your life, you can move toward manifesting your desires, resulting in a more positive attitude toward life. Daily gratitude increases your serotonin levels. This is your happy hormone, as discussed in Chapter 3. I believe like attracts like. By practicing daily gratitude, you increase your vibration, attracting higher vibrational circumstances to you.

Daily gratitude opens the door to more relationships and opportunities. I find that when people are not grateful, they stay stagnant and remain stuck in the same rut and the same routine. They transmit a low vibration. I refer to this as living in the hamster wheel. They have bad attitudes and often suffer from sadness and depression. They live in constant fear and remain unconnected to a source, almost like they are lost and have no purpose. Gratitude is a feeling of being thankful, a readiness to show appreciation for and to return kindness. Choosing to see the blessings all around us, big or small. By practicing daily gratitude, we raise our vibration and attract more blessings.

## Bringing Gratitude to Your Life

There are different tools you can use to remind yourself to practice daily gratitude. Some examples include giving thanks each day using a journal to list things we are grateful for. I like to tie this in with goal setting, writing my goals in the present tense as if I have already achieved them. As I write, I use all my senses and raise my vibration as much as I can.

I like to start my mornings by giving thanks to God and my Orishas, my guardian angels, and spirit guides. Then, I express gratitude for my immediate family, my husband, daughters, grandchildren, and then expand it to my parents, siblings, spiritual teachers, cousins, friends, and colleagues. My belief is that when we focus on the good, then good things continue to flow our way. When we focus on the negative, then negative things will continue to flow. God and my Orishas have been very good to me and my family. This is not to say that we have not been through some very difficult challenges, but they knew something better was coming. I have now learned not to attach myself to things. If it is not meant to stay, that is fine. Another opportunity will come. By being grateful, we are open to new experiences and opportunities. Like attracts like and when we are grateful and open, we will meet likeminded individuals with similar goals to us.

Our vibration increases when we are grateful. For example, let's say you are asking God or the universe for something and you are very grateful and happy. Your vibration is at a level nine or ten.

God's vibration is always at a ten. There is a very good possibility you will manifest your desire or wish. Now, let's say you are asking for something, but your vibration is only at a five because your emotions are not that of gratitude, but fear or disbelief. As stated above, God is at a ten vibration and chances are, the desire or wish will pass right over your five vibration and you will not see that which you asked. I believe this happens a lot and people then turn around and say the law of attraction is not real or is nonexistent. They are missing a key piece, which is their vibrational level at the time they are sending their wish or desire to the universe. We must work on ourselves, our beliefs, first. The other thing I have observed is that sometimes we think we are ready for something and we still have lessons to learn or we need to prepare ourselves. So, we will not get what we asked for because we are not prepared. God will not give you more than you can handle.

One of the messages I received during my experience with plant medicine is that music is one of the vehicles that increases our vibration. If you listen to music, that makes you happy, it raises your vibration. So, now as much as possible, before I ask God and my Orishas for my wish or desire, I listen to music that elevates me. It is very important when you listen to music, to pay attention to the lyrics. There are many subliminal messages in music, and they are not always positive. Don't get stuck in the beat alone, also listen to the lyrics. Some music installs fear, devaluates us as human beings and negatively impacts our mood. When I feel happy and I feel like my vibration is at a nine or a ten, I set my intention to God and my Orishas, and the vibration of the music carries my messages like a flying ship.

## The Wisdom of Letting Go

When the global financial crisis hit in 2007, we lost two businesses and four homes. We were forced to file bankruptcy. This was so devastating to me. So much work, time, and money invested and all lost. It seemed so unfair and I felt so sad and angry.

At that time, I had to choose which home to keep and give up the rest. I tried so hard to save all four and just fell deeper into debt and depression. I even contemplated suicide and thought if I die, at least my kids will be set. At that time, I had a decent life insurance plan. I remember I was driving on the freeway and thought if I just drive off the freeway, it will be an accident and my girls can collect the money and they will be okay. At that time, my daughters were in high school. As I contemplated driving off the freeway, my Aunt Silvia, my guardian angel, spoke to me and said how egotistical you are if you think money solves all your problems. Your daughters need you, not your money. Money comes and goes.

My Aunt Silvia was a very important part of my upbringing. She passed away in 2003 from breast cancer and she comes to me frequently. The thought of suicide immediately left me, and I began to cry and to thank her for snapping some sense into me. Then I asked God and my Orishas for forgiveness for even contemplating suicide and I thanked them for protecting me and never leaving my side. You see, they had a better plan for me and my family. If I had known that then, I would have never been so resistant to just letting everything go. Instead, I spent so much time and energy trying to hold onto something that did not serve me any purpose.

I look at my life now and I'm so thankful for a second chance without all that stress and pressure I had. You see, when I owned four homes and two businesses, I was also a full-time student and raising three teenage daughters. There was so much stress. My phone rang 24/7, I worked seven days a week, I was exhausted and could not see the light. I didn't know how to say no, so I said yes to everything and just worked myself into the ground. By losing everything, all that pressure was gone. It was a clean slate. This allowed me to rethink my current living situation. I learned how to say no and started putting some of my needs first. This was a period of reflection for me, a much-needed rest.

I currently live in a much nicer home than the ones I lost. I was able to pursue a degree as a holistic doctor. I had time to write this book. I work for a company that is dedicated to helping those in need and who have limited resources. This is where I belong. I am spending time with my family and enjoy my children and grandchildren. I am traveling to places I never imagined I would see and meeting wonderful people and friends all over the world. So many good things are happening to me, but had I not let go and continued to fight to keep everything I most likely would have ended up with a stroke or heart attack. By letting go and trusting in God and my Orishas, who had a better plan, I was able to reap the rewards.

## Simple Ways to Practice Gratitude

If you are not sure how to begin giving gratitude, start by setting your alarm fifteen minutes earlier and pray, meditate, and review your vision board and affirmations. When I have a long commute, I pray in the car. I say to God, my Orishas, and my guardian angels and spirit guides of the highest light, thank you for being with me and protecting me and my family. Thank you, thank you, thank you. Please continue to bless my children, husband, grandchildren, parents, grandparents, cousins, friends, and colleagues. Now, you may ask, why do you pray for your friends and colleagues? I do this because they are part of my family, too. If you think about it, as nurses, we spend as much time with our colleagues and friends as we do with our families. They are our families. So, I like to elevate their energy also because I spend time with them.

Another thing you can do is journaling. Write three things each day for which you are grateful. Practice this for twenty-one days and notice how your surroundings change. If you catch yourself writing something negative or thinking about something negative, stop yourself and reword it. Turn it into a positive statement. I always ask what lesson do I need to learn from this experience? That takes away some of the negative thinking. Besides journaling, prayer can also remind us to practice gratitude. During my prayers, I start by giving thanks. I feel like this helps me connect to the higher universal God. I look at it like we are his children; and, for those of us who have children, we like it when our children are grateful, and we don't like it when they have a sense of entitlement. I believe we are all energy beings and we go through life with vibrations of high, middle, and low. There are definitely things we can do to increase our vibration, such as practicing daily gratitude, prayer, meditation, laughing, and taking time to nurture ourselves; all examples of things we can do to raise the vibration.

Appreciate what you do have and what you have accomplished—even the difficult lessons. Remember what you learned from them. Whenever there is appreciation, there is duplication. For today's gratitude list, take five minutes to write three things for which you're grateful. If you're not sure how to start, begin by saying and writing, "I am so grateful for" or "I really appreciate" or "I am blessed because." If you find yourself thinking of only bad things that are happening, stop yourself because this drops your vibration, which is the opposite of what we are trying to accomplish.

When I feel like I am drifting into this negative thinking, I stop what I'm doing. I go outside, sit by a tree, look at the sky. Take a deep breath. If you have a pet, spend some time with your pet. If you have small children that make you laugh, spend some time with those children. If you are alone, you can YouTube videos of funny pets or children laughing. It is a really effective way of breaking that negative thinking. As soon as you feel happy again, continue with your gratitude list for the day.

## My Turning Point

This chapter commenced with me sitting on my couch feeling miserable. What changed me at that time? Tony Robbins came on the TV, and I was familiar with him because my Aunt Silvia gave me his book *Awaken the Giant Within* when I was fourteen years old. I loved my aunt so much that I figured anything she read had to be important. The infomercial was for *Get the Edge* and I pulled out my credit card and ordered it. I stopped crying, finished my ice cream, and said Tony will help me get back on track. This whole time my husband just smiled and said "I'm glad you got it. I hope he helps."

A couple of days later my package arrived. I was so happy. I opened it and my husband looked at me and smiled. He said, "You do realize that you actually turned thirty-one?" I said "What?!" I really thought I had just turned thirty. I said, "Why didn't you tell me when I was ordering the packet?" He said, "You looked so happy and you never do anything for yourself." We both laughed. I lost a whole year of my life and didn't even know it. I began listening to my CDs and writing my daily exercises and Tony delivered as promised. I began to change my thought process. I highly recommend researching Tony Robbins.

For my fortieth birthday I went to New Jersey and attended *Unleash the Power Within* personal development seminar. My friend and I got to go fire walking at this event. It was an amazing experience. Talk about facing your fears head on! Again, I highly recommend attending one of Tony Robbins seminars.

∼

# Your three action steps for this chapter:

1. Practice journaling three things you are grateful for daily. Try this for twenty-one days and see how opportunities come forward. Reflect on how doing this everyday has changed your life.

2. Write about one place you are thankful that you had the opportunity to visit, and why. When you are excited about that place you visited, see yourself in a new place and write it down. Use all your senses. Look at it daily.

3. Write down your morning prayer/gratitude prayer. What does it look like? Start incorporating it into your daily life.

When you are ready to take the next steps, head to the Appendices at the end of the book for more exercises that will help you practice daily gratitude.

∼

CHAPTER 5

# SUCCESS PATTERNS = RAPID RESULTS

~

"The key to success is to keep growing in all areas of life—
mental, emotional, spiritual, as well as physical."

**– Julius Erving**

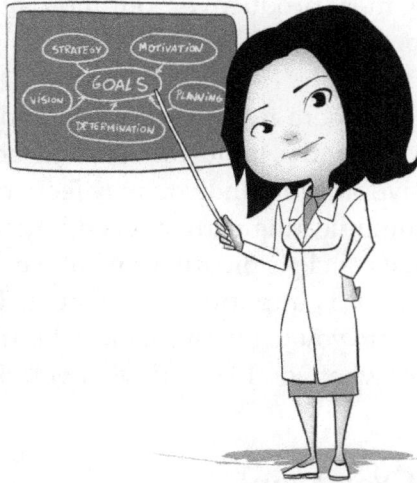

"See the world as your self. Have faith in the way things are.
Love the world as your self; then you can care for all things."

**– Tao Te Ching**

**H**ave you ever wished for more in your life but not been sure how to achieve it? Felt that there were things within your reach but not been clear on how exactly to attain them? The solution to how to reach that prize lies in your ability to set and achieve your goals.

Did you know people who write their goals down are 80% more likely to reach them than those who don't? Setting goals can help you focus your attention and achieve rapid results. Regular goal setting helps to organize your thoughts and allows you to perform at your best with a clear focus of what you really want. It increases motivation and encourages you to do your best. To successfully reach your goals you need a clear path and it is much easier to follow the steps when you see them in writing. Goal setting is the principle tool for helping you reach your true potential. As you achieve your goals, it will improve your self-confidence. You will have a positive attitude and find it easier to communicate with others. You will find yourself being more productive. Your thoughts and goals will become your actions.

Without a clear goal, there is a loss of focus and direction. You may have scattered thoughts, limit yourself, and lack motivation. It may cause a negative attitude, and you may feel unproductive and disorganized. Communicating with others might become difficult. Most of us don't have a clear picture of what we really want and what we don't want. It is important to define it. This takes work and time, but I implore you to take a couple of hours to write down a clear definition of what you like and what you don't like.

## Defining What You Want

I will share with you the way I like to organize my goals and set a clear intention. Now, this will change in time. Nothing is set in stone. As we get older, things will change. I like to categorize my goals, into areas such as spirituality, business and career, education and personal growth, money and financial well-being, friendships and community, and travel and creativity. This keeps me organized. I set achievable, measurable goals, short-term goals, and long-term goals. The important thing is to clearly define what you want. It is very important to balance work, rest, and play. I can't emphasize this enough.

Examples of my goals:

- **Spirituality:** I will pray and give thanks daily. I will meditate for fifteen to twenty minutes at least three times a week.

- **Health:** I will take my supplements daily and walk at least thirty minutes five times a week. I will choose healthier meals and practice mindful eating.

- **Career:** I will learn ways to perform my job more efficiently and delegate some of my tasks. I will continue to grow in my profession.

- **Finance:** I will set aside 10% of my check every pay period for new business ventures, travel, or to pay down debt.

Examples of defining what I do and don't like:

- **Spirituality dislikes:** I don't want to have limiting spiritual beliefs, for example, thinking there is only one way of praying. I don't like it when religions use fear as a way of hindering personal growth.

- **Spirituality likes:** Ability to learn about different faiths and how people from different countries worship. Knowing God loves me and encourages me to grow in faith and as a person.

Spirituality questions you can ask yourself: Do you feel connected to your God light source? Who are you? What is your mission in this life? Do you feel protected and guided?

- **Career and business dislikes:** I don't want to be stuck in an office. I don't want to work through lunch. I don't want to be without insurance or a paid vacation.

- **Career and business likes:** I want to have a flexible schedule. I want the flexibility of traveling to member's homes. I want excellent pay with great benefits.

Career and business questions you can ask yourself: Are you satisfied with your career or job? Do you wake up every morning eager to go to work? Are you doing what you love?

- **Money and financial well-being dislikes:** Living paycheck to paycheck, not having a savings account, not having an emergency fund, not being able to afford to travel.

- **Money and financial well-being likes:** Ability to travel, ability to generate income from known and unknown sources. I want to have a savings account. I want to have an emergency fund.

Money and financial well-being questions you can ask yourself: Are you satisfied with your income? What else can you do to generate extra income? When was the last time you received a raise?

- **Friendship and community dislikes:** I don't like to be taken advantage of. I don't like friendships that leave me drained. I don't like it when friends have negative attitudes or always see the glass as half-empty.

- **Friendship and community likes:** I like friendships that support me and empower me. I like it when friends see the glass as half-full. I like it when friends want to help and make a difference in the world.

Friendship and community questions you can ask yourself: Are you a source of inspiration for your family and friends? Are you a good example for those around you? Do you feel loved and supported by those around you?

- **Life partner and relationships dislikes:** Being controlled, poor listener, does not care what I think or how I feel. He does not value me as an individual.

- **Life partner and relationships likes:** He is flexible and well-balanced. He has great listening skills. He supports my goals and asks how I feel. I like setting boundaries and being flexible. He values me as an individual.

Life partner questions you can ask yourself: Does my life partner bring me peace and happiness? Do he/she support me in my vision and goals? Does my life partner bring out the best in me and do I bring out the best in them?

- **Education and personal growth dislikes:** Staying stagnant, believing that there is only one way to help our patients. Limiting beliefs that bring on fear.

- **Education and personal growth likes:** Knowing and pursuing different areas of healing. Continuing to learn ways to grow and improve myself.

Education and personal growth questions you can ask yourself: Regarding education, if given the time and resources, would you return to school? What would you study? And in terms of growth, in what areas of your life are you settling? If you achieve your goals how will you feel? What are you most afraid of? What do you wish you dedicated more of your time to?

- **Mind and body dislikes:** Not exercising, eating unhealthy foods, eating under stress, not honoring my body, not listening to the messages it gives me.

- **Mind and body likes:** Practicing mindful eating, exercising daily, acknowledging my feelings and releasing them in a healthier way, not using food as my scapegoat. I honor my body by listening to it. Getting seven hours of sleep and recharging. Incorporating yoga and meditation in my daily routine.

Mind and body questions, you can ask yourself: Is there an area that you would like to develop more fully? What is my why? If I continue doing what I do today how will it affect or benefit my life in one year?

- **Travel dislikes:** Not having enough money to travel, having a job that limits my vacation time.

- **Travel likes:** Traveling all over the world, having money to travel, having all the time I request to travel.

Travel questions you can ask yourself: Where have you always wanted to travel? What keeps you from traveling? What can you learn from other countries and cultures that will make you a better person?

- **Creativity dislikes:** Not thinking outside the box, having self-limiting beliefs.

- **Creativity likes:** Thinking outside the box, using my skills to generate passive income and coming up with new ideas that can help me, my family, and my patients.

Creativity questions you can ask yourself: Are you satisfied with your creative talent? Are you comfortable with change? What steps can you take to get out of your comfort zone?

# Living with Purpose

As nurses, we must balance our personal and professional life by having friends, family, and colleagues who love us and support us for who we are. They should lift our spirits and encourage us to pursue our goals and dreams, and we should do the same for them. You are here to live your life, so I highly recommend not wasting time and precious energy pleasing or impressing others. You are living your journey and they are living theirs. It is very important to pay attention to those with whom you surround yourself with. What is your work environment like? Who do you consider your friends? Ask yourself are they supportive of you?

I have learned it is okay to change my goals and not get so upset and stressed out when I don't meet them all. I've learned to be flexible, and sometimes I will delay some goals or even rewrite them. And it's okay to do that. I find setting goals keeps me more productive and I'm able to accomplish much more because I have a map that guides me, as opposed to just waking and seeing how the day goes without a map or a plan or any direction. It is like when you are driving to a place where you have never been. It's much easier to enter the address on Google Maps than just winging it.

When you have the map, you have direction and purpose. When you don't have the map, you waste so many hours and precious time looking for the address or purpose. I want to encourage you to set a couple of short-term and long-term goals. Review them daily. Don't get upset if you don't meet all of them. I guarantee you will meet most of them.

Finding an accountability partner for support can be very beneficial when you start goal setting. Finding a mentor is important too. Be honest and ask yourself, "What life goals do I avoid making and why?" I can guarantee it's either because there is fear or pain associated with the goal. Maybe you are telling yourself, "I can't function under structure." I would recommend changing the way you see the routine. Instead of looking at it as a chore, look at it as a step closer to obtaining your desires and goals. Start small by listing five personal goals and list two steps for each goal that will help you obtain it. That way, it doesn't seem tedious, but motivating.

I highly recommend journaling. Carry a small notebook with you and aim for thirty minutes a day. Have an ongoing conversation with yourself and reconnect with your inner self. Freely express your true feelings, wishes, and desires, with no judgment. If you are unsure what to focus on first, think about the successful patterns in your daily routine and ask yourself, "What area of my life makes me really happy?" Is it your health, your relationship, your career, your finances, or spiritual connections?

Now ask yourself what are the areas that need improvement and begin there. When you set a clear intention and define a clear goal, God's light source and the universe will make things happen. I can't emphasize this enough. As nurses, we are always giving and caring and leave our own needs to the end, if we ever even acknowledge our needs at all. It is important that you also take care of yourself and start defining some of your goals.

## Make Time to Make it Happen

When people ask me how I have done it, I always respond with, "The hardest part is starting." Once you decide to start caring for yourself and acknowledging your goals and desires, it is a nice ride. Please take a couple of minutes and write down some of the things you have always wanted to do or experience. Imagine money, time, and your relationship with spouses or children are not things you have to worry about at this time. This is about you. Now, read this over and over in present tense. When I read my goals, I also list incantations next to them. I will share some of them with you.

**Money:** "Bills are paid easily and quickly. I always have enough money to purchase what I desire. A constant flow of money is coming from multiple sources."

Now why do I put multiple sources of income? Because as nurses, we are experts at multitasking. We can function extremely well under crisis situations. We are creative, we have good hearts, and enjoy teaching and helping others. These are exceptional qualities with which to be gifted—and they also allow us to think outside the box. Think about it—how can you generate extra income? You could use this extra income to travel, go on spiritual retreats, pay debts, treat yourself to a nice getaway, go see Tony Robbins and go fire walking... That's what I did. Feed your soul, and get motivated to fulfill your goals and dreams.

**Travel:** "I am free to travel the world. Traveling feeds my soul."

Traveling improves your mood and lowers your stress levels. It allows you to learn about other cultures. Traveling broadens your perspective and opens up creativity.

**Career:** "I continue to grow in my profession."

Setting goals holds us accountable and keeps us on a timeline, allowing us to continue to grow as individuals and not remain stagnant. When you write your goals and review them on a daily basis, you are letting your subconscious mind know you are ready to receive them. When you have a clear purpose and understanding of what you do and don't like, situations and opportunities will present themselves to you. You may be wondering why it's important to list the things you dislike. The reason is because it's easier to define what you really want by eliminating what you don't like.

~

# Your three action steps
# for this chapter:

1.  List three goals you would like to achieve and write down two steps you can take now to reach those goals.

2.  Write down your greatest motivation in life and the goals that will leave you feeling the most fulfilled. List three barriers or fears that hold you back in obtaining your goals and list one or two things you can do to remove or decrease those barriers or fears.

3.  It's essential that you review your goals regularly. Keep them in front of you and look at them daily or list them on your vision board.

When you are ready to take the next steps, head to the Appendices at the end of the book for more exercises that will help you set and achieve your goals.

~

# CHAPTER 6

# VISION 2 REALITY

~

"Whatever you hold in your mind on a consistent basis is exactly what you will experience in your life."
— **Anthony Robbins**

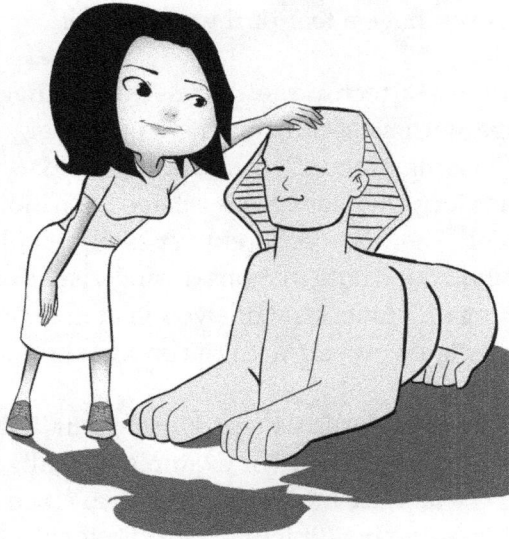

"If you don't have a clear vision of where you want to be, you probably aren't going to get there."
— **Ti Caine**

What if I told you there was a strategy that is simple enough to do every day, but powerful enough to help you meet the Dalai Lama or travel the world? Our mind is so strong that it can create our reality and fulfil our dreams. When we use the power of our mind through the technique of visualization anything is possible.

Visualization can aid in manifesting your dreams and wishes, helping you to reach your highest potential. Visualization can build confidence and improve your performance. Visualization techniques have helped me fulfill my dreams and wishes.

Without visualization techniques, you can feel as though you are stagnant and not getting anywhere. You may lack confidence and limit yourself. Or maybe you see visualization as wishful thinking? You might even have a fear of the unknown.

Visualization is a technique that uses the imagination to help people cope with stress, fulfill their potential, and activate the body's self-healing process. Visualization can assist with pain relief, allergies, anxiety, phobias, stress-related conditions, and personal development. There are different types of visualization, such as guided visualization, affirmations during visualization, and vision boards. Using affirmations while you visualize can program your brain to associate yourself with the end goal.

Try to use all your senses when you use visualization techniques. Make it as real as possible. For example, visualize yourself at the beach, near a waterfall, in a forest, or at a park. See it clearly in your mind, and imagine how it looks, sounds, smells, tastes, and feels. Practice using a vision board to improve finances, plan trips, or further your education. You can list anything you want. The sky is the limit as this is your vision board. Vision boards provide you with a daily reminder of your dreams and goals. These are your dreams and goals so don't hold back.

## Practical Visualization Technique

I'd like to share with you a visualization technique that can help you if you are experiencing stress or feeling overwhelmed.

Find a quiet area where you will not be disturbed for ten to fifteen minutes. Lie down in a comfortable position, close your eyes, take a couple of deep breaths. Inhale slowly through your nose, and exhale slowly through your mouth. Do this three times.

**Visualization to overcome stress:** Now, imagine golden rays of light over the top of your head, extending down your body, covering every inch of you. Imagine this light is coming from the universal God, the universal light. As the light covers you, you have a sense of warmth, love, health, and internal peace. This light knows exactly what requires attention at this time and will heal that area for you.

**Visualization for illness:** Visualize as above, then imagine your T cells, which are one of your body's defense mechanisms. They hunt down and destroy cells that are infected with germs or have become cancerous. Imagine the T cells are gathering the disease, illness, unhealthy emotions, and clumping it in a container, and the golden light is destroying the containers you have collected. Now you feel stronger, healthier, and happier. Then, imagine your thymus gland developing more T cells so that you are always ready and protected.

Finish by imagining yourself strong and healthy and give thanks for this amazing healing. This can take ten to fifteen minutes. You can practice it any time you want. For example, when I am having a difficult day at work, I practice it during lunch.

If you're thinking, "I don't know how to visualize," or, "I don't have time," as with meditation, there are tools to help you. There are guided visualizations and YouTube videos that help with making vision boards. I prefer to do my visualizations in the morning and start my day with a positive outlook. You may ask yourself, "What if I'm not doing it right?" As with meditation, there is no right or wrong way. Only you know what your visions and desires are, so you cannot help but do them correctly. There is no need to put pressure on yourself. Write down all your goals and desires and read them daily. If you're wondering what visualization has to do with nursing, consider the bigger picture. When we are excited about where we are in life, we can't help but provide better care for our patients and family.

## Bringing Your Vision to Life

Using visualization can improve your performance and confidence. Let me share with you a couple of my visions that have come true.

About four years ago, I decided to move my pictures and images from my journal to a full-size vision board and hang it up in my room next to my bed, where I could see it every morning and every night. I read them when I wake up, and I read them when I go to bed. Some of the things included were a picture of the sphinx, the OM sign, angels, a healing center, Ganesh and Buddha (which I associate with India), a family on a cruise boat, and a woman meditating. Some of the words I cut out and posted were Barcelona, Australia, Ecuador, practice self-healing, simplify your life, author, everything is in divine and perfect order right now, dream it, plan it, and do it. I can say with great joy I've had some awesome opportunities. I got to go to Mexico and experience plant medicine with the shamans. I went to India and participated in the 33rd Kalachakra Initiation with the Dalai Lama. I traveled to Peru with wonderful people and met amazing shamans. I traveled to Egypt and had an amazing experience connecting with Sekhmet. I currently rent a space with amazing healing practitioners that offer many healing services.

Several years ago, I had just started a new job and was still on my probation period when my aunt called me and asked me if I wanted to go to India. One of the ladies that was supposed to go on the trip with them had canceled. I remember this conversation with my aunt like it was yesterday. I said, "I just started new job and I'm on probation. I don't even have vacation time to go." She said, "It does not hurt to ask." When she said that, I remembered part of my vision board and going to India was on there. So, the next day, I called my boss and I said, "I have the opportunity to go to India and attend the 33rd Kalachakra Initiation with the Dalai Lama." My heart was racing, and I was praying, "Please say yes!" Guess what she said? Yes!!!! I thanked her so much. She said she had the opportunity to listen to the Dalai Lama once and it was an incredible experience.

I went home that night and looked at my vision board and cried and thanked God over and over again for this amazing opportunity. I have traveled to London and been to Stonehenge. I went to New Jersey and New York and went fire walking with Tony Robbins. In February 2019, I went to Australia to attend a retreat with Ultimate 48 Hour Author, who is assisting me in publishing this book. Never in a million years did I ever think I would leave the U.S. I am a high-school dropout, and I had three daughters by the time I was twenty-one years old. Visualization, prayer, meditation, connecting to our universal God and my Orishas really work. I am living proof. I encourage you to try it and see what happens.

My dreams are to travel. What are yours? Whatever they are, gather a bunch of magazines, cut out pictures, words, phrases, goals, anything that you desire. Then, paste them on your vision board and put this in your room where you can see them day and night. Use all your senses. Picture yourself on a plane, looking out and imagining what it will be like when you land, for example, in Hawaii. Imagine yourself walking out of the plane and being greeted by the hula dancers, receiving a lei, the smell of the lei, the pretty view, the pretty ocean. God and the universe have a funny way of allowing these opportunities to present themselves.

~

# Your three action steps
# for this chapter:

1. Let's start by making your first vision board. Be sure to list things that always make you smile and happy. Write five big dreams that have not come true yet. The key is to look at them frequently, daily if possible, and see what happens.

2. Sit in a quiet area and practice a couple of guided visualization techniques. Be sure to use all your senses with this exercise.

3. List ways in which you can incorporate visualization in your daily routine.

When you are ready to take the next steps, head to the Appendices at the end of the book for more exercises that will help you practice visualization and make your dreams a reality.

~

# CHAPTER 7

# ULTIMATE BALANCE

~

"When we develop the heart chakra, we begin to influence the surroundings with our spiritual presence. When we develop the communication chakra, we begin to influence the country with our spiritual presence. When we develop the seventh chakra, we begin to influence the world with our spiritual presence without doing anything."
**– Swami Dhyan Giten**

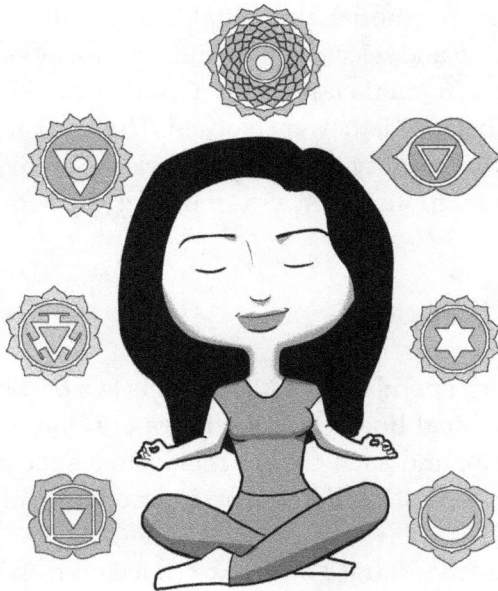

**M**y Aunt Silvia introduced me to chakras when I was a young child. She told me that we are not just made of a physical body but an energetic body also and just because we can't see it, doesn't mean it doesn't exist. She said your energy centers are your chakras and she taught me how to practice guided mediation to balance the chakras and what the colors represent. I would like to share this with you and my hope is that it helps you as much as it has helped me.

What are chakras and why are they so important? Chakras serve as collection and transmission centers for both subtle and metaphysical energy and concrete or biophysical energy. Chakra balancing is beneficial in transforming your weakness into strength, allowing you to find your inner strength. It will allow you to express and release emotions in a healthy manner.

The word chakra in Sanskrit means "spinning wheel of light." Chakra balancing provides you with a faster and greater ability to heal your physical, emotional, mental, and spiritual issues. It can assist in balancing and releasing unhealthy non-supportive patterns. It will also bring mental clarity and a more focused mind. When chakras are unbalanced, they are blocked. This can cause weakness, irritability, or an inability to express or release emotions. Blocked chakras may lead to illness, stress, and foggy and forgetful mind.

## The Seven Chakras

Each chakra corresponds with and connects to a particular location within the physical body. Every chakra is related to a specific endocrine organ, and each chakra relates to a specific frequency, base, color, and sound. I will give a basic description of each chakra.

**First chakra—Muladhara:** The base or root chakra is located at the base of the spine, between the anus and the genitals. It governs understanding of the physical dimension and is the energy center through which we experience flight or fight. It externalizes as a spinal column and glandular system. Its color is red and the sound associated with this chakra is LAM.

Affirmation: "I am." I am grounded. I am safe. I am secure. I am healthy.

An imbalance in this chakra, might show through symptoms such as constipation, diarrhea, urinary tract infection, lower back pain, sciatica, impotence, pain in your legs, knees and feet, obesity, or anxiety. Positive qualities of this chakra are stability, vitality, prosperity, patience, and career success. Associated stones are hematite, red jasper, black onyx, black tourmaline, and black obsidian.

**Second chakra—Svadhisthana:** The sacral chakra is located in the lower abdomen. It governs attitude and relationships, sex, and reproduction. It externalizes as the sexual organs, ovaries for women, testes for men. Its color is orange and the sound is VAM.

Affirmation: "I feel." I am creative. I am adaptable. I can enjoy the pleasures of life.

An imbalance in this chakra could lead to sexual or fertility problem, isolation, hip, or sacral iliac joint problems. Positive qualities include joy, creativity, adaptability, sensuality, pleasure, and sexuality. The associated stones are carnelian, red jasper, amber, orange calcite, and copper.

**Third chakra—Manipura:** The solar plexus chakra is located above the naval and below the breastbone. It governs emotional sensitivities and issues of personal power. It externalizes as the pancreas and adrenals. It governs the action of the liver, spleen, stomach, gall bladder, and aspects of the nervous system. Its color is yellow and the sound is RAM.

Affirmation: "I do." I can do anything to which I set my mind. I am powerful and use power wisely.

An imbalance in this chakra could result in digestive issues, kidney or liver problems, rage, diabetes, ulcer, chronic fatigue, or low self-esteem. Positive qualities are confidence, charisma, humor, mental clarity, and leadership. The associated stones are yellow jasper, tiger's eye, citrine, amber, and golden calcite.

**Fourth chakra—Anahata:** This is the heart chakra located in the chest. It governs the heart, blood, and circulatory system and influences the immune and endocrine system. It externalizes as the thymus. Its color is green and the sound is YAM.

Affirmation: "I love." I am loving and lovable. I am deeply compassionate.

An imbalance in this chakra may cause us to lose touch with our emotions and relationships and be unable to express ourselves or create. We may lack energy and stop advancing on our life path and our journey. An imbalance may lead to asthma, allergies, immune disorders, or heart and lung problems. Positive qualities include love, trust, healing, compassion, and connection. Associated stones are rose quartz, green aventurine, malachite, and peridot.

**Fifth chakra—Vishuddha:** This is the throat chakra, located in the throat. It governs the lungs, vocal cords, and metabolism. It externalizes as the thyroid and parathyroid gland. Its color is light blue, and the sound is HAM.

Affirmation: "I speak." I know my truth and I share it. I am guided by the deepest purpose.

An imbalance in this chakra can possibly result in thyroid or hearing problems, teeth or gum issues, tonsillitis, stiff neck and shoulders, TMJ, or fear of speaking. Positive qualities include truth, purpose, expression, artistry, service, and communication. The associated stones are turquoise, blue agate, aquamarine, and blue topaz.

**Sixth chakra—Ajna:** This is the third eye which is located between the eyebrows. It governs the lower brain and nervous system, the ears, the nose, and the left eye. It externalizes as a pituitary gland. The color is indigo or purple and the sound is OM.

Affirmation: "I see." I am intuitive and follow my inner guidance. I always see the big picture.

An imbalance in this chakra may cause vision problems, migraines, nightmares, sleep disorder, sinus issues, or lack of intuition. The positive qualities are good vision, intuition, dreams, perception, mental clarity, and stability of mood. The associated stones are amethyst, lapis lazuli, kyanite, pearl, and sapphire.

**Seventh chakra—Sahasrara:** This is the crown chakra which is located on the top of the head. It governs higher learning, parts of the immune system, parts of the hypothalamus, and the right eye. It externalizes as a pineal gland. The color is white, also seen as violet or golden and the sound is OM.

Affirmation: "I understand." I am intelligent and aware. I am one with everything.

An imbalance in this chakra could manifest as Alzheimer's, confusion, sadness, mental illness, depression, or apathy. Its positive qualities include unity, wisdom, awareness, intelligence, and bliss. The associated stones are crystal quartz, moonstone, selenite, pearl, amethyst, and labradorite.

# Bringing Your Chakras into Balance

Balancing chakras can be accomplished through guided mediations, yoga, biomagnetism, Reiki, energy healing, movement, and with the aid of crystals. I would like to share with you two exercises you can practice in clearing chakras.

**Exercise one:**
Sit in a chair, rest your hands on your thighs, have your feet firmly touching the ground, and close your eyes. To open your chakras, breathe in seven times and breathe out seven times. Do this three times. Now picture your legs are like the roots of a tree. One root is going down the center, one root is going down your right leg, one root is going down your left leg. Now you are grounded and connected to Mother Earth, Pachamama. Next, picture a golden light coming from heaven from the light source. This light is filled with unconditional love and healing properties. Imagine this light entering through your head and going down your body as it gently flows through you. It is bathing every single cell in your body, filling it with life, love, and boosting your immune system.

As the light flows through you, not only is it filling you with unconditional love and healing, but it's filling you with strength, courage, self-love, and giving you creativity. It awakens your intuition. It is picking up feelings of fear, anxiety, stress, fatigue, nervousness, anger, sadness, disappointment, and resentment, and releasing it to Mother Earth, where she has the power to destroy it.

As the light from above is going through your chakra centers, imagine each center lighting up with the following colors. When it reaches your root chakra, located at the base of the spine between the anus and the genitals, visualize a glowing red sphere. Feel grounded and secure. Now let go of any fear.

When it reaches your sacral chakra, located in the lower abdomen, visualize a golden orange sphere. Feel your creativity and let go of any guilt.

When it reaches your solar plexus chakra, located above the naval and below your breastbone, visualize a golden yellow sphere. Feel your personal power and let go of any self-doubt.

When it reaches your heart chakra, located in the chest, imagine a green sphere. Feel unconditional love and let go of any sorrow.

When it reaches your throat chakra, located in your throat, visualize a light blue sphere. Feel how easily you express your needs and desires and let go of any suppression of the truth.

When it reaches your third eye, located in between your eyebrows, visualize an indigo sphere. Feel peace and stillness and let go of any misunderstandings.

When it reaches your crown chakra located on the top of your head, visualize a purple sphere. Feel the connection to a higher source and let go of any lack of direction. Now return to your breath and give thanks for this wonderful gift of self-healing.

**Exercise two:**
This exercise uses crystals—you can refer back to the chakras and choose the crystals associated with the chakras on which you would like to focus, or you can choose to focus on all your chakras.

Lie down in a comfortable position and place the stone in the chakra position associated with it. Now take three deep breaths, inhale slowly through your nose, and exhale slowly through your mouth. Picture the color of the chakra on which you would like to set your intention. Picture the color getting brighter and brighter, turning counterclockwise, energizing this chakra. You can use the affirmations listed under the descriptions of the chakras. You can imagine any physical elements associated with this chakra as healed. When you are finished with the healing, close a chakra by turning it clockwise one time. This exercise can be done daily, or you can choose one chakra to focus on per week. Chakras draw the healing energies of the crystals into your body and then release this energy into your aura.

When finished with the crystal clearing chakra exercise, cleanse the crystals by leaving them under moonlight, or in sunshine the next day. Alternatively, you can clean them with ocean water or use incense to smudge them. Clearing your chakras, will improve physical, emotional, mental, and spiritual issues as each chakra is responsible for a certain part of your body and mind. By keeping your chakras aligned and radiant through regular practice, you can optimize the higher vibrations of each chakra.

## How Your Chakras Affect Your Health

Each chakra has a specific relationship to areas of your health and body. When blocked, it can cause illness, pain or discomfort. Here's a short summary of the ailments associated with each of the chakras:

- **A blocked root chakra** may manifest as lower back pain, sciatica, anemia, constipation and digestive disorders.
- **A blocked sacral chakra** may manifest as stomach ulcers, heartburn, obesity, nervous disorders, liver, spleen, or gall bladder problems.
- **A blocked solar plexus chakra** may manifest as menstrual pains, prostate problems, hip-joint pain, or kidney problem.
- **A blocked heart chakra** may manifest as coronary illness, cold and lung infection, asthma, allergies, or high blood pressure.
- **A blocked throat chakra** may manifest as tonsillitis, speech defects, shoulder and neck pain, and thyroid problems.

- **A blocked third eye chakra** may manifest as migraine, headaches, sinus problems, or middle ear problems.
- **A blocked crown chakra** may manifest as headaches, immune weakness, depression, and sleep disorders.

≈

# Your three action steps
# for this chapter:

1. First, let's name and define the seven chakras. Identify the color associated with each and think of ways you can begin to incorporate these colors into your life.

2. Practice clearing your chakras. Choose either exercise one or two and journal your experience with it. Include the benefits of balancing your chakras in your journal.

3. Utilize chakra balancing to improve your health. When doing the above exercises, was there a chakra or chakras that you felt needed more healing? What steps can you take today to balance your chakras?

When you are ready to take the next steps, head to the Appendices at the end of the book for more exercises that will help you balance your chakras.

≈

# CHAPTER 8

# *BEYOND GUILT*

~

"Guilt is to the spirit what pain is to the body."
**– Elder David A. Bednar**

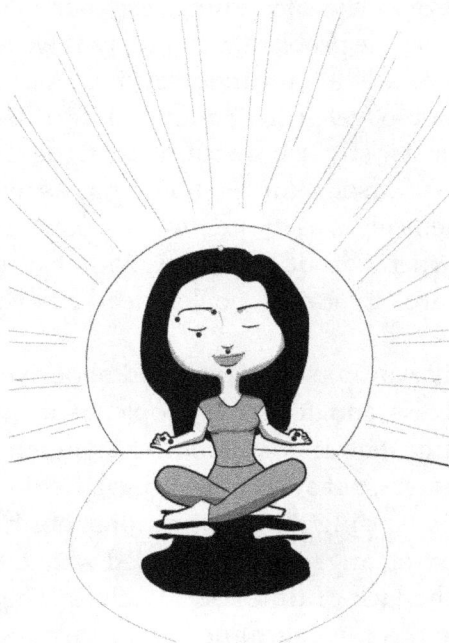

"Guilt isn't always a rational thing… Guilt is a weight that will crush you whether you deserve it or not."
**– Maureen Johnson**

When my daughters were in elementary school my life was in a phase of competing demands. I had three beautiful young girls to take care of. At the same time my career was going well and in my commitment to my patients I felt like I was pulled in different directions. This was a challenging time for me personally as two of the elements that I value most highly were at times competing with each other, both wanting and needing my attention. The consequence for me was many anxious moments of feeling the burden of guilt.

Guilt is a nagging part of your conscience that says that you have fallen short of a certain standard to which you want to live up to. Guilt can serve as an internal warning system that helps us identify unethical behavior. The problem with nurses is we feel guilty about everything—especially about underserving. As a fellow nurse, I encourage you not to feel guilty about making self-care a priority. Self-care can decrease stress, burnout, and fatigue. Think about it as an investment in yourself. Nurses should pay as much attention to taking care of themselves as they do to their patients. Your patients will recognize when you do, and they will also recognize when you don't take care of yourself. So, let's lead by example.

A feeling of guilt can make you feel bad about yourself and can cause anxiety, stress, and, for some people, depression. As nurses, we may feel guilty about not spending as much time with our children and spouses, not attending extracurricular activities with our children or attending family functions, not having as much patience, and getting angry and frustrated with our children and spouses about the lack of time for ourselves. These are some of the common themes my colleagues and I discuss during lunch. How is it that we are so good at caring for everyone else, but when it comes to our personal life, we tend to drop the ball more than once? I know, for me personally, this was very difficult when my daughters were in elementary school.

# Letting it Go

It is important to ask yourself, why am I holding on to guilt? When we criticize ourselves, we are less motivated, and this can lead to anxiety and depression. I have learned in my career to allow myself to feel and acknowledge my emotions so if I need to cry, I cry. If I am angry, I verbalize my anger. I don't internalize my emotions any longer, as this can lead to physical and mental illness. I encourage you to spend time exploring and acknowledging your emotions either through writing in a journal, meditation, or seeking out peer or professional support.

By releasing guilt, we can feel at peace, forgive ourselves, meet our needs, and show ourselves compassion and self-love. We can stay physically and mentally healthy and learn to establish healthy boundaries. By getting enough rest, eating healthy meals, and by attending to your needs, you can be a better nurse. Increased anxiety and stress can come from holding on to guilt, causing overeating, feelings of overwhelm, loss of boundaries, and becoming a people pleaser. Harboring feelings of guilt can show up as depression, emotional outbursts, increased levels of cortisol causing weight gain, increased muscular aches and pains, headaches, back pain, indigestion, and a compromised immune system, which can eventually lead to a mental or physical illness.

When I was in Mexico, I participated in a ho'oponopono retreat. It is the practice of reconciliation and forgiveness. Ho'oponopono is translated to "to put to right, to put in order or shape, correct, revise, adjust, amend, regulate, arrange, rectify, tidy up, make orderly or neat." We were encouraged to take full personal responsibility and then the healing process began. Guilt was seen as an opportunity for learning, as an opportunity for reconciliation and to take responsibility for ourselves, allowing us to forgive ourselves and have self-acceptance. We all gathered in a circle and let go of any guilt and began our new journey free of any prejudice.

Guilt is one of the hardest areas in my life with which I have had to work. I have read books, gone to retreats, attended seminars, met with shamans, spiritual healers, and still, this guilt has been with me since I was a child. Gradually, over the years, I have become much better at not feeling guilty about things. Now think of your own needs. As nurses, what are some limiting beliefs you are carrying inside? This may stem from childhood. We want to treat ourselves with the same level of uprightness that we guarantee others.

I would like to share with you an exercise that can be used to release some of these limiting beliefs. It is an emotional freedom technique, known as EFT. It is a self-help technique that involves tapping near the end points of "energy meridians" located around the body.

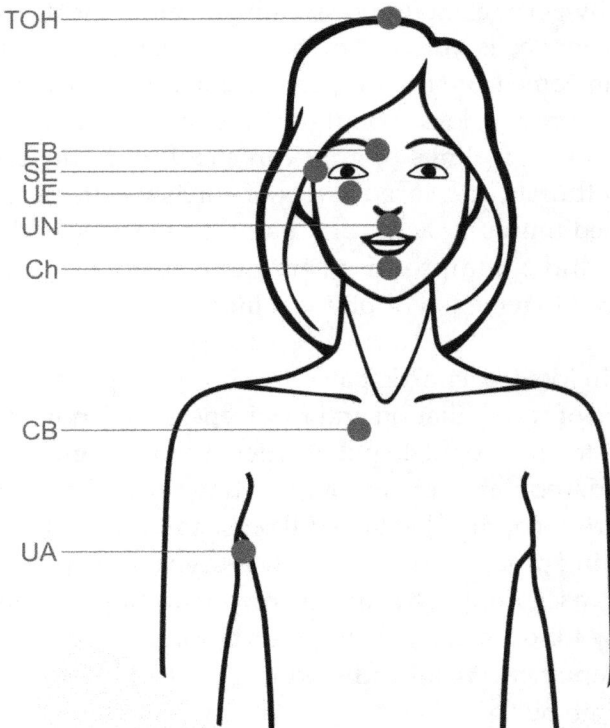

To do this exercise, you focus on the limiting belief you have. Prepare a tap. You can tap on both sides of your face at the same time. While continuing to focus on the memory, gently tap with your fingers four to seven times on each of the following locations: top of head, inside of the eyebrow, outside of the eye, under the eye, under the nose, on the chin, on the collarbone, under the arm, and on the inside of the body about four inches below the armpit. Continue to focus on the memory and repeat the tapping procedure, tapping on each point in succession. When you notice a shift, adjust your focus and start over. You can use affirmations such as, "Even though I feel I can't (name your fear) I completely accept myself. I see myself as a powerful person who can master anything. I am capable of doing anything I desire." Affirmations should always be used in present tense.

## Eating for Balance

Another common area of concern for us as nurses is stress eating. We tend to eat our emotions. As discussed in Chapter 2, stress and anxiety can lead to overeating. One effective exercise to incorporate is starting a food journal asking yourself the following questions:

- What did I eat today?
- What was my emotional state just before eating?
- What was my emotional state after eating?
- What was my energy level before eating?
- What was my energy level after eating?

The right foods can be incredibly healing. Here are some of the best foods recommended to balance your chakras:

**First chakra, Muladhara:** root vegetables like carrots, potatoes, radishes, beets, strawberries, and cherries.

**Second chakra, Svadhishthana:** melons, mangos, oranges, salmon, papaya, and sweet potato.

**Third chakra, Manipura:** grains like cereal, flaxseed, yogurt, sunflower seeds, grapefruit, and squash.

**Fourth chakra, Anahat:** spinach, kale, broccoli, and celery.

**Fifth chakra, Vishuddha:** water, herbal teas, and blueberries.

**Sixth chakra, Ajna:** blackberries and grapes.

**Seventh chakra, Sahasrara:** sacred incense, smudging, fasting, and detoxifying.

In Chinese medicine, certain foods are associated with emotions. For example:

**Sour food** is associated with the liver and the gall bladder. Emotions enhanced by eating sour food is anger. Emotions reduced by eating sour food is thought.

**Bitter food** is associated with the heart and small intestine. Emotions enhanced by eating bitter food is joy. Emotions reduced by eating bitter foods are sadness and worry.

**Sweet food** is associated with the spleen and the stomach. Emotions enhanced by eating sweet food is thought. Emotions reduced by eating sweet foods are fear and shock.

**Pungent food** is associated with the lung and the large intestine. Emotions enhanced by eating pungent food are worry and sadness. Emotions reduced by eating pungent foods is anger.

**Salty food** is associated with the kidneys and bladder. Emotions enhanced by eating salty food is fear and shock. Emotions reduced by eating salty foods are joy.

If you are thinking, "Stress, burnout, guilt, and physical, mental and emotional drain are all part of my daily job as a nurse." Yes, they are. I agree. As nurses, we are responsible for our patients and their families. Most of us in the nursing career have issues with codependency. But this should not mean that we are so exhausted that we do not make time to take care of ourselves. Please don't put your needs to the end, because in that way they will never be met.

I had to retrain my mind. I learned that if I take care of myself, I acknowledge myself, I love myself, then I have more to give. My glass will be full versus half filled. This takes time and practice. But I guarantee when you switch your mentality, everyone around you will respect you and your patients will want to model you, and they themselves will practice self-love. My definition of self-love is acknowledging your needs, taking care of yourself, and making sure you are eating healthy and exercising regularly.

A study at Stanford University in California stated spending time in nature reduces the level of anxiety and stress and improves sleep. Taking time out in nature, practicing gratitude, and connecting to God daily are all valuable ways to replenish and care for yourself. Some people define self-love as being selfish, egotistical, and uncaring. That's not my definition. You may feel guilty when putting your needs first. This is the way most of us as nurses think and feel. However, I have learned throughout my career that putting my needs first allows me to give more. Patients know when we are not feeling well. We don't do our jobs to the best of our abilities. By taking care of ourselves, we show up to work feeling energized, physically and mentally prepared to help our patients and their families.

~

# Your three action steps for this chapter:

1. Write down any feelings of guilt you may be harboring. There is no right or wrong here. Spend as much time as you need.

2. List ways in which you can start practicing self-love and self-care today. Some examples may include connecting to God, reading a book, going for a walk, talking to a good friend, or soaking in the tub. I like to add two cups of baking soda, two cups of Epsom salt and a handful of Himalayan salt and soak in the tub for twenty minutes.

3. List some resources or people you can contact when you are feeling bad or guilty or need a pep talk.

When you are ready to take the next steps, head to the Appendices at the end of the book for more exercises that will help you let go of guilt.

~

# CHAPTER 9

# UNLOCKING CONNECTION

~

"Words have energy and power with the ability to help, to heal, to hinder, to hurt, to harm, to humiliate, and to humble."

**– Yehuda Berg**

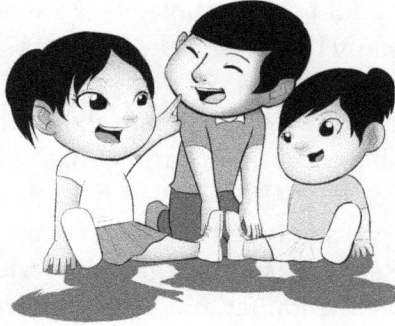

"Anything that annoys you is teaching you patience. Anyone who abandons you is teaching you how to stand up on your own two feet. Anything that angers you is teaching you forgiveness and compassion. Anything that has power over you is teaching you how to take your power back. Anything you hate is teaching you unconditional love. Anything you fear is teaching you courage to overcome your fear. Anything you can't control is teaching you how to let go."

**– Jackson Kiddard**

I remember at a hospital I worked at, my colleagues and I were discussing how important it was to express how we felt. Most of us had way too many patients to take care of and not enough help. It made us feel really upset because the patients complained we were not doing our jobs. In the thirty years I have been in health care there have been so many changes. Technology is now a big part of our health-care system but unfortunately it has taken away some of the face-to-face time with our patients. Now more than ever having the right communication strategy is so important.

A common theme with nurses is, we believe we are not entitled to express our feelings, or to ask others for what we want. We think we should always please others and meet their needs and expectations. This was discussed most during our lunch break and is one of the leading causes of nurse burnout.

Effective communication can lead to a happier life full of self-expression and freedom. Saying how we feel is something we can learn how to do. Many times, we believe others should know how we feel even though we have not disclosed our feelings, and we become resentful because they don't care about our needs. Learning why we have trouble expressing our feelings can go a long way.

An inability to express yourself can lead to suppressed emotions and physical illness, such as weight gain, hypertension, insomnia, digestive disorders, mental fatigue, stress, and alcohol and drug abuse. When communicating, we should avoid words that have negative connotations, such as can't, won't, and no. Negative connotation words provoke a negative, emotional response.

Effective communication is very important in the nursing field. The words we speak have energy and power. When we speak, we can help to encourage or to hurt. By having good communication skills, we can express our feelings in a healthy manner. It is important in setting boundaries and learning how to say no. We can also offer hope to our patients, family, and friends.

# Different Ways to Communicate

Active listening is one of the most important communication skills you can have. Active listening involves paying close attention to what the other person is saying, asking clarity questions, and rephrasing what the person said to ensure understanding.

Nonverbal communication is using your body's language. For example, eye contact, facial expression, hand gestures, and tone of voice. Having a relaxed stance, with arms opened and legs relaxed, sends a very different message than being closed off, with arms crossed and sitting or standing in a very rigid position.

When you use phrases such as "I understand" you show empathy to others. Empathy is defined as the ability to understand and share the feelings of another. Having an open mind, being flexible, being open to listening and understanding the other person's point of view, will produce an honest, productive conversation. If respect is conveyed, people will be open to communicating with you and expressing their true feelings.

It is very important that we give and receive feedback. When giving feedback, it should also include praise. When receiving feedback, look at this as an opportunity for growth. As nurses, we are constantly growing and evolving. Some differences in communication styles between doctors and nurses are that nurses communicate in broad, narrative, descriptive styles and doctors communicate using pertinent information as in, "What is the problem?"

A healthy team functions effectively by having open communication, clear direction, a respectful atmosphere, and shared responsibility. Some of the misunderstandings in hospitals in which I have worked occurred because some nurses were given patient assignments with high-acuity levels, and some were not. This created an unhealthy atmosphere, because the responsibilities were not shared equally. Barriers in communicating at the workplace may include personality differences, generational differences, personal values, and expectations. This is why having unit meetings is very important. When you get to know your colleagues, you understand what their values and expectations are. It makes for a better working relationship.

## Speak Out

As nurses, we are role models to our patients, family, and friends. During my time working in health care, I have worked in some areas where I felt I could not express my feelings and concerns to the higher-ups. This really affected my self-esteem and made me feel powerless. This caused me great frustration and conflict at work. I felt as if I was in survival mode. I needed to work, and I needed the money. This was early in my career, and I did not really think outside the box. I didn't think about choices at that time. If you are working in a place where you are oppressed and not empowered, not given breaks or meals, have inadequate staffing ratios, limited supplies to perform your job in a safe manner, or you or your colleagues are humiliated or defamed, I highly encourage you to quit this job. It is not a healthy environment. Your environment should allow you freely to express how you feel. And if you need help or more education, you should be encouraged to pursue your goals and grow as an individual, so you feel alive and full of energy.

When you work in a healthy environment and are able freely to express your wants and needs, you can't help but perform at 150%. Your confidence and self-esteem will grow, and you will radiate a high vibration that will benefit all those around you. As nurses, you are powerful and an inspiration to those around you, so lead by example.

## Communicating Effectively

Communication affects everything we do. Which is why is it so important to express how you feel. Communication comes with a responsibility to be truthful to ourselves and others. Lack of communication may have been a result of force of habit through upbringing, or may stem from a single traumatic incident, either known or locked deep in the subconscious. We are better nurses when we have mastered the power of effective communication. As nurses, we have a multitude of responsibilities when it comes to patient care. We relay and interpret information among physicians, caregivers, family members, and patients. Developing good communication skills will assist us in providing the best care and patient outcomes possible.

What are some of the things you can do to communicate more effectively? Here are some examples of different communication interaction you may encounter during your workday.

**Nurse-to-nurse managers communication, including administrators.** I like to write key notes down on a piece of paper when I communicate with nurse managers and administrators. They are like providers and have a full plate, attending unit meetings, and overlooking multiple projects, so I want to be direct and get to the point. Now as I have evolved in my nursing career, if I have a concern or a problem, I will bring it up, but then I also have two or three solutions to the problem or concern. I feel nurse managers and administrators respect the fact that I actually took time to think about the problem, and the solution to the problem.

**Nurse-to-nurse communication.** In nursing school, I was taught and continue to use SBAR. S stands for situation, B stands for background, A stands for assessment, and R stands for recommendation. This tool is very effective during shift changes. Effective nurse-to-nurse communication can significantly improve patient care.

**Nurse-to-provider communication, including supporting staff.** Providers are out there rounding, so they need the specifics about the patient condition, or any changes that recently occurred. The SBAR can also be utilized here.

**Nurse-to-patient communication, including his or her family.** I was always taught you don't get any special brownie points by using medical terminology with your patients. The aim is that the patients and their families understand what is going on with their health care. They need to be included and treated as a person, not a number. So, I like to pretend I am treating my grandparents, mother, father, brother, sister, or children, and offer the same love and care to my patients.

This is where we can use our active listening skills. You will be surprised how much key information the patients and their families will give us if we just take a moment to listen. If I have to teach a member about a medication, or how to monitor his/her blood pressure, or blood sugar, I give a brief explanation of what I am doing, and why I am doing it. I like to use a teach-back method, asking patients to repeat the information in their own words. It is always important to assess the patient's ability to understand the instructions. This is where including the family is key. I like including the family members because they will assist in caring for the members when they are home.

Developing effective communication is essential to releasing our pent-up emotions. Can suppressed emotions cause you to become overweight? The answer is yes. Food triggers our pleasure and reward center in our brain, so we feel better. Unfortunately, this creates an unhealthy behavior that ends up creating a cycle of feeling bad about yourself after you binged. What you really need is a hug. Why a hug? Because hugs increase oxytocin, which reduces stress in the body. If you don't want a hug, spend some time petting your pets. Oxytocin is a hormone that promotes feelings of love, bonding, and well-being.

As I stated earlier words are very powerful and they carry energy. As nurses and health-care professionals sometimes we encounter low vibrational energies, so there is a prayer I would like to share with you. I use this prayer when I feel weighed down, exhausted and am not thinking clearly. I call upon God to dissolve all holds that are holding me back at this time. This includes holds I have on others, holds others have on me and those I have placed upon myself, whether they be to people, places, things or belief systems. My belief is that every moment we come in contact with another person we are exchanging energy.

~

# Your three action steps for this chapter:

1. Practice making your nurse communication more effective.

2. Research some communication styles, such as nonverbal communication, active listening, showing compassion, cultural awareness, and written communication.

3. When dealing with conflict at work or at home, write down how you feel and come up with a healthy way of expressing your emotions with your colleagues and family, working through your feelings.

When you are ready to take the next steps, head to the Appendices at the end of the book for more exercises that will help you communicate effectively.

~

# CHAPTER 10

# *DO YOUR OWN THING*

~

"Life is too short to wake up with regrets. So, love the people who treat you right. Forget about those who don't. Believe everything happens for a reason. If you get a chance, take it. If it changes your life, let it. Nobody said life would be easy, they just promised it would most likely be worth it."

**– Paulo Coelho**

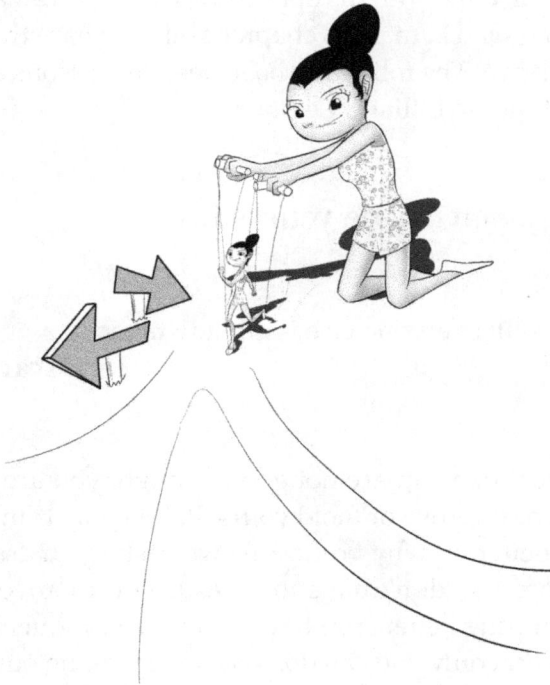

"Life is a song—sing it. Life is a game—play it. Life is a challenge—meet it. Life is a dream—realize it. Life is a sacrifice—offer it. Life is love—enjoy it."

**– Sai Baba**

As I shared with you earlier in this book, I am a high school dropout. I finished my GED at 16 and then went on to pursue my high school diploma and my nursing education. I have been wanting to write a book for over ten years, but you know what stopped me? Fear. Most of the people I work with and my family and friends have been encouraging me to write a book for years, but I had doubts. What can I possibly offer? Who really wants to listen to my story?

I know what it is to have doubts echoing through your mind. I understand what it is to feel unsure and vulnerable. I am grateful life has presented me with the opportunity to learn valuable lessons for embracing who I am. This chapter seeks to share those lessons so you can thrive. The following have been my lessons and for this reason I call them "Lillian's Lessons."

## Lillian's Lesson #1: Be yourself.

"Be yourself; everyone else is already taken."

**– Oscar Wilde**

When you feel like you are not good enough, you are constantly trying to fix or improve or mold yourself. You may think everyone else does it better, so why bother? News flash—you are your own unique being. You don't have to measure up to anyone else, so erase this limiting belief. You have your own uniqueness to offer to the world that only you can do. Instead of looking outward, look inward and develop your God-given gifts, and I guarantee no one can do it better than you. I take great pride in being different and embrace it and give thanks daily for it.

## Lillian's Lesson #2: Practice being true to yourself.

By not embracing your uniqueness, you may continue living your life for someone else and fulfilling their hopes and wishes, not yours.

## Lillian's Lesson #3: Be creative.

When you ignore your creative side, it may feel like living in a prison where you become stagnant, alone, depressed, and harbor feelings of resentment.

## Lillian's Lesson #4: Prioritize your passions and gifts.

They will give you liberation and freedom. Ask yourself, what are you passionate about? My belief is that in this life we are all teachers and students, so what is your special gift? What will you teach others? I encourage you to look deep inside and find that special gift you possess. Only you can nurture it and develop it and share it with the world. Don't allow a state of fear to hinder your special gift. Fear is crippling and a way of controlling the masses, but you are unique and original.

## Lillian's Lesson #5: Be your own boss.

Instead of spending time, energy, and money trying to be like someone else, why not invest that time, energy, and money on yourself? What would you do differently? What risks would you take if money or time were not a factor? You are not part of the masses that are being controlled.

With these lessons in place I was able to clarify my purpose and overcome my fears. Fear can stop you doing things that allow you to move forward and achieve your goals. It can also stop you from expressing your uniqueness because of what others might say or think. Fear is a limiting belief. It will not allow you to grow or take risks. Don't deny yourself your universal gift of free choice.

## Go Beyond Fear

With my fears to one side I set myself the goal to write a book, this book. But how would I do that? My experience is in nursing, not in writing books. Well, I took my own advice and got help. I attended an Ultimate 48 Hour Author workshop in California hosted by Natasa and Stuart Denman. As I sat in there in the introductory session, I said to myself, "This is it." Natasa asked for a volunteer, and my arm shot up so fast. For those of you who know me, you'll know I don't like speaking in front of people. I turn red, and I mumble, and I just get so nervous. But, my gut said, "Just do it," so I did.

Natasa chose me, and, long story short, here I am writing my heart and soul and sharing with you my life experiences, not because I am in any way an expert, but because I have fallen so many times and gotten up so many times. I want to motivate you to try your own thing. Who knows, it might even be writing your own book. I hope I can help you avoid some of the pitfalls I have experienced through my own life experiences. I encourage you to do things that bring you joy and happiness. It won't even feel like work. When you wake up in the morning and you are passionate about what you are doing, time goes by so fast.

Change your thinking process. It is so easy to get caught up in negative thought and attitude because of everything we see on TV and social media. Most of it, in my opinion, is 90% fear-provoking. It also provokes anger, anxiety, and sadness. I choose not to get caught up in that. I know there are good people who really want to help, and that as a whole, people are good. My belief is by installing fear you limit a person's ability to become independent and think for themselves. It's a way of manipulating the masses. Most people don't take risks because of fear of the unknown.

## Explore Your Talents

Most nurses are good at multitasking. We are creative, independent, and intelligent. I always encourage my friends and colleagues to do their own thing. This does not mean you have to quit your job. What I mean is there is always a way to generate extra income. Pursue your talents and gifts because there is definitely a feeling of empowerment when you do your own thing, whether it is a hobby, teaching, or starting your own business.

There are countless opportunities for nurses to branch out into other areas. We can become consultants, educators, life coaches, and wellness coaches. We can own and operate assisted living homes, foster homes, home health agencies, wellness spas, or beauty spas. We can write books and blogs. You name it. I am planting the seed for you to look at your creative side and see what you can do. If you choose, you can generate extra income, share your talent and create more freedom in your life.

In my career, I have owned and operated a couple of businesses. When I was an LPN and taking my prerequisites for my RN, I lived in Arizona and would buy clothes in California and resell them at the Community College. I made decent money. This helped me pay for some of my classes. As a registered nurse, I owned and operated Mobile Physicals where I would go to the local high schools and perform sports physicals. This was a good business because it was a mobile service. I went to the high school, set up shop at the gym, and performed my sports physicals. It was flexible, and it generated good income. I owned and operated two assisted living homes. I did this while I was in school pursuing my master's and family nurse practitioner degree. This was a very rewarding business. I really enjoyed it. It allowed me to send my daughters to private college prep high schools.

When I moved to California, I owned and operated an importing business that allowed me to travel and meet wonderful people in India, Egypt, and Peru. I was able to purchase essential oils, perfumes, clothing, and crystals, and resell them in the United States. It allowed me to learn about different cultures and grow as a person.

I most recently started Synergy Holistic Care & Wellness. I work with my eldest daughter Lillian, who is a nurse aesthetician. Our goal is to incorporate Eastern and Western healing practices. Some of our services include:

- homeopathy
- herbal medicine
- detox
- biomagnetism therapy
- essential oils
- energy healing therapy
- collagen induction therapy
- facials
- microcurrent
- nutritional counseling
- lifestyle coaching
- Reiki therapy
- microdermabrasion
- B-12 injections
- microneedling
- dermaplaning
- peels

I have also loved writing this book. I hope it inspires you to tap into your creative talents.

When I owned and operated my businesses, I kept my day job that provided me benefits and a steady income. My businesses allowed me to provide a better life for my children and now grandchildren. It also gave me the freedom to travel and experience life through a different lens. I could donate to some of my favorite charities, one of them being House of the Lord, an orphanage located in Mexico, and give back to the homeless population by providing clothing and food.

In the future, my plan is to open a fund where I can assist individuals who have been victims of domestic violence and provide them with scholarships so they can pursue their degree and follow their goals and become strong, independent individuals who break the cycle of abuse.

## Overcoming Doubts

You may say to yourself, "I don't know how to be creative." I can share with you I also struggle with being creative. My whole family is creative. I feel like that gene skipped me. Some of the things I have done to practice being more creative is traveling. When I travel, I see the world through a different lens. When I traveled to Peru, I saw three-year-old's who were speaking five languages, and I asked myself "Why are we so stuck on English only?" What a limiting belief. I wish I could speak five different languages. I wish my daughters could speak five different languages.

The second thing I did was start taking classes at the local community college. They have so many choices, such as photography, making natural soaps, baking cakes, developing your own website, learning how to play instruments, budgeting, creative writing. You name it, they have it. I encourage you to challenge yourself and sign up for a class that allows you to express that creative side of you. The key is stepping outside of your comfort zone.

What if you don't know what you want to do? If you do not have a clear image of your God-given gift, you may pray, meditate, visualize, and be open to receiving messages. I always say, "God, and my Orishas, my angels and guardian angels, and my spirit guides of the highest light. Please bring me clarity. Please protect me and guide me and help me," and then I'll list my problem or concern. My belief is we have free choice. If we don't ask for help, they cannot help. Try it and see what happens.

An activity you can practice to awaken your creativity is walking, as it can stimulate the free flow of ideas. Meditation also produces a state of relaxation and alertness, an ideal space for creativity to bloom. You could also play music, as studies have shown that listening to classical music produces short burst of creativity. Learn how to knit or try an adult coloring book. Put your brain in the state of relaxed alertness required for the free flow of ideas. Practice relaxation techniques such as yoga, massage, deep breathing, or have a warm shower or bath. These all cause mental relaxation, allowing your brain to move into a creative state.

As I've mentioned, fear can stop you from fully experiencing life. If you're afraid to step outside your comfort zone, there are some actions you can take to decrease fear. First, I would recommend investing in yourself. It is a great way to get rid of fear. By educating yourself, you prepare yourself. Get the information or knowledge you need. Learn as much as you can about it.

Another way to decrease fear is by asking for the help of a mentor who has walked down the path you are pursuing. They can be a key resource in guiding you to reach your goal. Find out his or her formula for success. I also like using peer pressure. When I announce my intentions to the world, it puts pressure on me to do it. I have a tendency to procrastinate, and by announcing my intent, it gives me accountability. Since I take pride in my word—I got this from my grandfather—then I follow through. I surround myself with people who will push me to overcome those fears.

Networking is also key to getting yourself and your talents out there. Find like-minded individuals who support you. You can download the app Meetup, which provides you with resources in your community and online, or you can join Facebook groups.

Now, with technology, everything is at the tip of your fingers. The use of visualization, meditation, and prayer can eliminate fear.

Most importantly, don't forget about having a positive attitude. Keep trying. Don't give up. Sometimes you have to take breaks. That is okay. The key is getting back up to do it and being persistent and determined, two of my favorite words. Keep your eye on the target, the goal, the end result.

~

# Your three action steps
# for this chapter:

1. Make a list of some of your hopes and wishes.

2. Write down your special gifts and how you can incorporate them in your life. If you are not sure what they are, try to remember what brought you joy and happiness when you were a child. What did you love doing? What comes easy to you? What are some of the compliments you get from others?

3. Find ways to connect with others, including networking to expand your knowledge and base.

When you are ready to take the next steps, head to the Appendices at the end of the book for more exercises that will help you uncover your gifts.

~

# CHAPTER 11

# HEAL YOURSELF

~

"Nourishing myself is a joyful experience, and I am worth the time spent on my healing."

**– Louise Hay**

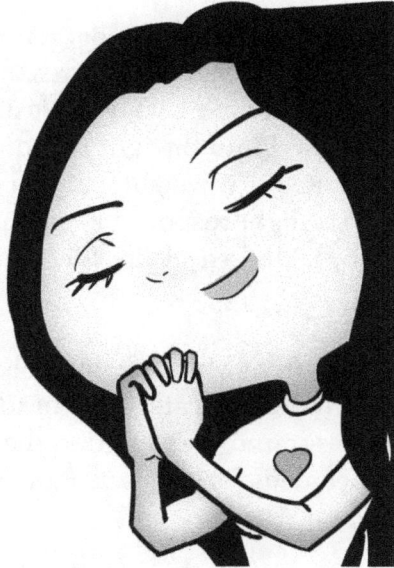

I would like to introduce you to some alternative healing therapies that can aid you in self-care and self-healing. Healing therapies offer a different approach to self-healing. Using these therapies improves the body as a whole, enhancing your spiritual, emotional, mental and physical health. Healing therapies such as relaxation techniques and breathing exercises have been known to lower blood pressure, decreases stress on the cardiovascular system, improve psychological stability, and increase activity of the immune system resulting in less susceptibility to illness.

Healing therapies bring emotional calm and increase alertness and energy. When left unchecked, stress, fatigue, and burnout often lead to other complaints, such as high blood pressure, depression, obesity, and physical illness. When we are stressed, our levels of lactate increase. This lowers the flow of the blood and oxygen throughout the body and increases the levels of cortisol. Elevated cortisol over a sustained period produces glucose, which can result in increased blood sugar and obesity.

You can lower your cortisol levels by getting the right amount of sleep, relaxing, exercising, and decreasing stress. When you experience a stressful situation, your levels of adrenaline increase. This is known as the flight or fight response, and it can cause restlessness and irritability, weight gain, anxiety, and headaches. When your flight or fight response kicks in you can lower your adrenaline levels by taking a deep breath, meditating, and practicing yoga.

Some of the therapies from which you might benefit are listed below. I've placed them under the categories of touch and movement, medicinal therapies, mind and emotion therapy, relaxation, and breathing, and included a brief description of each.

## Touch and Movement Therapies

- **Massage** is a hands-on technique that can be applied across the entire body or in specific targeted areas. It is used to promote relaxation, increase circulation, remove tension, reduce stress and anxiety, and improve sleep.

- **Reflexology** is a type of massage that aims to relieve nervous tension by applying finger pressure to targeted areas of the body, in particular the feet. It is also known as zone therapy. Massaging certain points in the body releases energy blocks and stimulates your natural healing powers.

- **Acupuncture** involves inserting a needle at certain points on the body with the aim of balancing the energy. Originating in traditional Chinese medicine, it is commonly used today for the treatment of pain, stress relief and overall wellness.

- **Acupressure** involves a practitioner applying pressure using the thumbs or fingertips with the aim of clearing blockages to allow life energy to flow freely through the body. It focuses on the same points of the body which are stimulated in acupuncture and is used primarily for the relief of tension or pain.

**Here's a simple acupressure technique used to relieve stress and anxiety:**

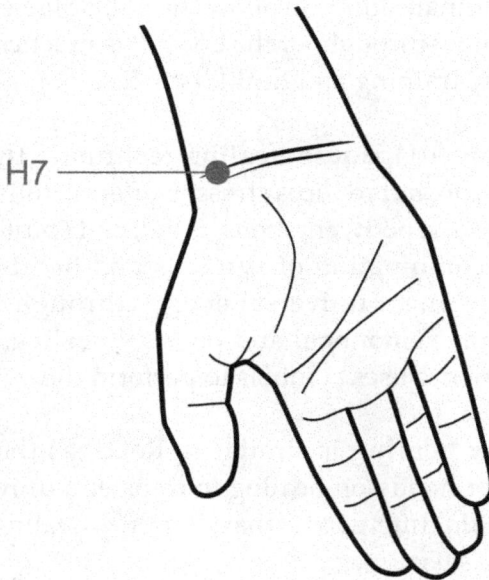

H7

Start from the wrist, measure down with three fingers. Where your third finger touches the middle of the wrist is the acupoint. Take your thumb and apply firm pressure to this point until you feel mild discomfort. Only apply enough pressure to interrupt the normal blood flow, but not too much that it causes pain. Hold this pressure point and gently knead your thumb in a tight circular motion for about two minutes. Do this to both wrists and you will feel your anxiety descend immediately. (Credit: www.modernreflexology.com)

- **Biomagnetism** uses special magnets placed on certain areas of the body to regulate and maintain the optimum pH. According to Dr Luis F. Garcia, the aim is to "attain bio-energetic balance in the human body; the state of natural health, known as homeostasis." Through this therapy you can reestablish homeostasis and eliminate pH imbalances so that the body can heal itself.

- **Tai chi** is based on the principle that the mind is integrated with the body. It teaches control of movement and breathing to generate internal energy, and enhanced mindfulness. The ultimate aim is to allow the chi, or life energy within us, to flow throughout the body. It is practiced for both its defense training and health benefits.

- **Reiki** is a Japanese healing technique that promotes relaxation and reduces stress. It offers a holistic approach, treating the body, emotions, mind, and spirit. Practitioners use a combination of symbols and hands-on healing, transferring a universal energy through the palms to encourage emotional and physical healing. In Reiki, the practitioner uses symbols to perform the healing.

- **Energy healing** is similar to Reiki, as the healer uses palm or hands-on healing to transfer a universal energy. The main difference is that in energy healing there are no symbols used.

- **Yoga** uses a combination of breathing techniques, exercise, and meditation. It can improve overall health and happiness and cultivate discernment, awareness, self-regulation, and higher consciousness in the individual. It is a group of physical, mental, and spiritual practices, performed using postures called asanas.

## Medicinal Therapies

- **Naturopathic medicine** uses natural, non-invasive practices to work with the inherent self-healing process by identifying and removing the underlying cause of illness, instead of trying to eliminate or suppress the symptoms.

- **Aromatherapy** uses plant-derived aromatic essential oils to enhance both physical and psychological well-being. It can help to relieve a wide range of ailments including stress-related problems such as insomnia, depression, anxiety or tension. For example, eucalyptus helps with burnout and stress, frankincense clears the mind, coriander increases confidence, rose aids love and compassion, and cedarwood is grounding and prevents the absorption of other's negativity.

- **Homeopathy** is a medicinal system based on the law of similars. The theory is, that if a substance can trigger similar symptoms to those suffered by the patient, then a minute dose of the same substance will encourage the body to overcome the illness. The remedies simulate the body's natural ability to cure itself.

- **Bach flower remedies** are used to reduce negative emotions and restore the natural balance between the body and the mind. They are made from spring water infused with the essence of wildflowers, with the addition of a grape-based brandy as a preservative.

# Mind and Emotion Therapies

- **Biofeedback** is a technique that is used to help you learn to control some of your body's involuntary functions, such as your heart rate, and help you gain a greater awareness of your psychological functions. It can assist in the treatment of migraine headaches, chronic pain, and high blood pressure.

- **Meditation** is a process of quieting the mind in order to spend time in thought for relaxation, or religious and spiritual purposes. The goal is to attain an inner state of awareness, intensify personal and spiritual growth, and achieve a mentally clear and emotionally calm state.

- **Creative visualization** is the process of generating visual and mental imagery, with the aim of transforming the visions into reality. It can be performed with your eyes closed or open and is used to minimize pain, heal the body, modify emotions and alleviate negative feelings, such as anxiety, stress, sadness and low moods.

- **Music therapy** is the use of music to improve health and functional outcomes. It can help to improve a range of physical and mental health complaints, including emotional and behavioral problems. It has also been used to help relieve stress and treat depression and anxiety. It is often used to help elderly clients deal with memory loss associated with Alzheimer's disease and dementia.

- **Chromotherapy (or color therapy)**, uses light in the form of color to balance energy within the body. It works within the body and mind on all levels—emotionally, spiritually, mentally and physically.

- **Neuro-linguistic programming (NLP)** is based on the idea that there is a connection between our neurological process, language, and behavioral patterns learned through experience, and that these can be altered to help us achieve specific goals in life. It can be used for personal development, phobias, and anxiety.

## Relaxation and Breathing

- **The 4-7-8 breathing** exercise is a fast and simple conscious breathing technique. It can be done almost anywhere and once you have mastered it you can perform it an any position, but it's a good idea to sit with your back straight to begin with. The following instructions are taken from wellness expert Dr Andrew Weil's website (https://www.drweil.com) where you can also find an instructional video.

Place the tip of your tongue against the ridge of tissue just behind your upper front teeth and keep it there through the entire exercise. You will be exhaling through your mouth around your tongue; try pursing your lips slightly if this seems awkward.

1. Exhale completely through your mouth, making a whoosh sound.
2. Close your mouth and inhale quietly through your nose to a mental count of four.
3. Hold your breath for a count of seven.
4. Exhale completely through your mouth, making a whoosh sound to a count of eight. This is one breath.
5. Now inhale again and repeat the cycle three more times, for a total of four breaths.

Note that you always inhale quietly through your nose and exhale audibly through your mouth. The tip of your tongue stays in position the whole time. Exhalation takes twice as long as inhalation. The absolute time you spend on each phase is not important; the ratio of 4:7:8 is important. If you have trouble holding your breath, speed the exercise up but keep to the ratio of 4:7:8 for the three phases. With practice, you can slow it down and get used to inhaling and exhaling more and more deeply.

- **Pranayama** is a formal practice of controlling the breath to maximize the flow of prana ("life force") in your body. It is used to enhance overall health and give you more energy.

On my travels I have learned some of these therapies and have worked out over time which work best for me. I encourage you to find the therapies that resonate most with you and to develop your own personalized self-care plan and implement it into your daily routine.

~

# Your three action steps
# for this chapter:

1. List some self-healing therapies you would like to incorporate into your daily life.

2. What does your self-care plan look like?

3. Research further self-healing therapies and self-care therapies.

When you are ready to take the next steps, head to the Appendices at the end of the book for more exercises that will help you utilize healing therapies and practice self-care.

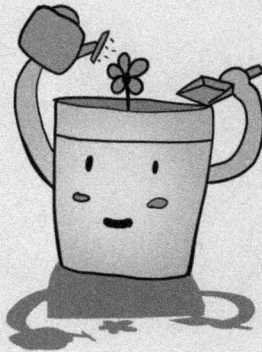

~

# CHAPTER 12

# MY JOURNEY WITH AYAHUASCA, KAMBO AND BUFO

~

"I took a walk in the woods and came out taller than the trees."

**– Henry David Thoreau**

Throughout this book I have shared many insights and knowledge gained through a culmination of life experience, learning and reflection to help you nurture and care for yourself. My journey so far has taken me to many places—both physically and spiritually—in my search for answers on how to lead a better life. In this final chapter, I want to share the story of my time at a healing retreat I attended in October 2017, in Tepoztlán, Mexico (this city is also known as The Mystic Mountain Village) which was an amazing and life-changing experience for me.

I feel blessed to have had the opportunity to attend this retreat firsthand as it is not something that many people are able to do. I am sharing my experiences and the life lessons I learned, in the hope that it gives you a glimpse of what is possible and what lies inside us all.

# Retreat Day 1

### Ayahuasca #1

We were all gathered in a living room area. There was approximately thirty of us, of all ages and from all walks of life. We all had that nervous look except for two or three that had participated in ayahuasca ceremonies before. The shaman and her assistants sat in the front where there was an alter with candles and incense burning. There were musical instruments such as drums, guitars, flutes and rain sticks. The shaman explained that once we took ayahuasca we were to sit up for at least thirty minutes and we had to stay in the living room for direct supervision. Her assistant then passed out small buckets for all the participants. They then demonstrated the recommended way to vomit into the bucket. Each participant had their own sleeping bag and a small pillow.

They dimmed the lights and all we had were the candles that were lit in the alter. We then formed a line to drink ayahuasca. I remember as I was in line thinking, "Oh man this is it—no turning back now." I was also forming a protection circle around me (I do this by imagining a white light surrounding my whole body). When I got to the beginning of the line I knelt down and held the bowl with ayahuasca close to me and asked, "Who am I?" I drank it down. The taste was a little bitter but not bad at all. I went back to my spot grabbed my bucket and covered my eyes with a blindfold, as the shaman had suggested we blindfold ourselves so that it was an internal process.

I felt a little nauseated and was nervous, and I remember asking myself "What are you doing?" but then something incredible happened. I saw lights everywhere—bright colors like I have never seen before and they were all connected. Then I saw myself in front of a huge tree. This magnificent tree was lit up by all the bright colors and it was so peaceful. Everywhere I looked I saw splashes of yellow, blue, green, red and orange. I remember thinking how lucky I am and then out of nowhere I heard my husband Victor say

"I can't breathe" and all the bright colors turned black and gray and it started raining. I began to cry and feel sadness for him because he was in a lot of pain. My heart hurt for him and I began to vomit.

I spent the rest of the night hurling and crying, I could not stop. In the distance I heard the shaman say we have to separate them she is picking up his emotions. Then for a brief second I saw an image of my mother saying you're too strict with your daughters you're causing them too much stress. We stayed in the living room until three or four in the morning and then everyone who wanted to go went off to their rooms and the rest stayed in the living room.

# Retreat Day 2

## Kambo #1

I signed up for kambo as recommended by the shaman. Kambo is a traditional medicine used by South American tribes which comes from the secretion of an Amazonian frog Phyllomedusa bicolor, also known as the giant monkey treefrog. It is meant to clear your emotions in a physical way and to prepare we were asked to drink two liters of water. A ceremony was held outside where they set up two chairs and we formed a line. It was soon my turn and the assistant asked me if I had drunk my two liters of water to which I responded "Yes." He then gave me my bucket and asked me to focus on something. I chose to focus on the tree. He then took a wooden stick and got some of the kambo and burned seven dots in my arm applying kambo in each dot. That was a little painful, but nothing compared to the hurling I was about to experience.

My whole body felt swollen—my eyes, my mouth, my whole body. I kept on staring at the bucket I had never seen so much vomit and I am a nurse. The assistant kept telling me focus on the tree, so I did even though it lasted thirty minutes or so. It felt like hours. I was in pain, the most intense feeling. Every part of me felt achy and swollen and I vomited like never before. After I was done, I felt a sense of relief and a light sensation came over me. I then got up very slowly as I was feeling very weak, I picked up my puke bucket who during this retreat became a good friend and went to my room and slept for a couple of hours. I said to myself, "I am never, ever doing that again."

## Bufo #1

For this ceremony we all sat outside, and the shamans put some sleeping bags on the grass. Bufo comes from the Bufo alvarius toad which inhabits the areas surrounding the Colorado River. Its glands secrete venom which contains psychedelic substances which is smoked. The shaman and her assistant are at your side and you are then asked to inhale slowly while they count up to fifteen. I can honestly say all I remember from this experience is flying high past this universe I lost total control of my body. My eyes closed, and I became flaccid.

I remember the assistant lying me down and I remember I had my hands closed and I was pounding the floor and I could hear myself saying "release, release, release." Then I disappeared. I became small particles that floated off into the universe. I became part of the universe. Then I said, "I surrender" and my hands opened, and I felt an overwhelming emotion. I then began to cry and felt so much pressure taken off my chest. A great sense of peace came over me. I lay with my arms open and palms facing up. I was open to the universe. I went back to my room and slept some more.

In the evening we all gathered in the living room and the shamans gave talks and asked who wanted to share their experience. At first everyone was shy and quiet, but it only took one person to start and then everyone wanted to share. Some participants struggled on a physical, mental, emotional, or spiritual level and had general confusion over what they experienced with ayahuasca, kambo and bufo.

## Ayahuasca #2

As we did on day one, we all picked our spot, but this time they put my husband across the room, with literally twenty people between us. The alter was set with candles, music and incense. This time I sat next to a young boy who could have been my son to my right and to my left a lady a little older than me. I was forty-five at the time. Again, most of us had that look of fear because the shamans said to us ayahuasca gives you what you need not what you want, and each day will be different.

We got up formed a line and I set my circle of protection as I waited in line.

When it was my turn, I knelt down and held the bowl with ayahuasca close to me and asked, "Who am I?" I then went back to my spot grabbed my bucket put on my blindfold and sat up and waited.

I heard a female voice ask me "Do you want me to heal you?"

I responded "Yes," and I immediately felt a rush. The best way to explain it is every single one of my cells was examined, I mean every single cell in my whole body was thoroughly examined.

Then she said, "I touched every one of your cells and your problem is not physical but emotional. Do you trust me?"

"Yes" I replied, and she said, "Do you want me to heal those emotional scars?" I said, "Yes please."

I began to yawn and take deep breaths and she said, "I am releasing trapped emotions. I am healing your scars."

I said, "Thank you so much." Then I heard another female voice say, "Do you know who I am?" I replied "Yes," and she said, "I have been waiting for you."

I said, "I am sorry I deviated" and she replied, "It's okay you are here now." She then said, "Your question was who is Lillian—who are you?"

"Yes." I replied. She said, "You are who you are, a being of pure light."

I then felt for the very first time in my life an overwhelming sense of unconditional love like I have never ever experienced. She said, "You see the person next to you?"

"Yes" I replied. "He is also a being of light. You are him and he is you. Do you understand?"

"Yes." I replied. "So, you see there is no right or wrong it is all one."

She asked me to open my hands, and spread my fingers, then said, "Do you feel me?" I felt energy in both my hands, an overwhelming energy. "Now place your hands on your heart." I did as she asked. "I am inside of you. Stop searching outward and start searching within yourself for I am there." I felt so much unconditional love and gratitude I kept saying, "Thank you, thank you, thank you, I understand."

Then Darwin, a gifted musician who sang his inspirational songs during our retreat, began to sing and play his guitar and she said, "Open your hands and spread your fingers. Feel the vibration of the music. Do you feel it?" I replied, "Yes."

When the song was finished, she said "Now place your hands on your heart. Music heals the soul." I said, "I understand. Thank you, thank you, thank you." Then she took me by the hand, and I felt like I was six years old we walked together. She talked to me about my ancestors and took me to other dimensions where all that exists is light and vibrations, and universal love and peace like I have never experienced. There was a feeling of protection, a feeling of being safe and loved. I could hear myself speaking in another language it was not English or Spanish or any language I recognize here on earth. While I was talking to who I believe is God another female voice greeted me and said, "I just wanted to say hello." I said "Hello," and I didn't hear from her again. I feel it was one of my Spirit Guides.

This was truly a wonderful experience. But before it all ended ayahuasca said you have to do all three days of kambo it is clearing your liver and your pancreas. I had just told myself earlier today I would never ever do kambo again.

# Retreat Day 3

## Kambo #2
Where to begin! I was really not looking forward to doing kambo again but ayahuasca said I needed it, so I waited in line drinking my water and holding my precious bucket. I then decided to let go and relax knowing this would help heal my emotional scars. The assistant lit the wooden stick put kambo on and inserted seven more dots going across forming a cross symbol. I immediately felt a sense of purging. My whole face and body felt so swollen, it felt ten times worse than the first day.

The assistant kept saying focus on the tree I kept on looking at the bucket. I could not believe all the stuff I was vomiting it was not bile or blood it was not food I have no Idea what it was, and I have seen a lot of vomit in my life. When I finished, I felt a great sense of relief and could hardly walk to my room. When I got to my room I laid in the fetal position and I just remember thinking my intention for kambo was to heal all my emotional scars that have limited my beliefs. As I laid in bed, I had a sense of tingling and heat, a stronger sensation then the day before. It took me a lot longer to recover.

## Ho'oponopono therapy #1

In the evening we had our therapy session and we were introduced to ho'oponopono. We all sat in a circle and the counselor would pick a participant and ask what experience they had the night before. One gentleman stated his parents did not protect him when he was a child and the counselor asked him to look around the room and pick his mother and his father out. The counselor and shaman asked us all to participate in the ho'oponopono therapy.

He chose me to play his mother. The irony was that I was told by my mother that I was too overprotective on day one of ayahuasca, yet I felt like I always dedicated more time to my career than to my children and that brought on a great sense of guilt.

We role-played and I said what the counselor asked me to say to the gentleman. Ho'oponopono states "to put to right, to put in order or shape, correct, revise, adjust, amend, regulate, arrange, and rectify." There are four simple steps to this method they are Repentance, Forgiveness, Gratitude and Love.

We were encouraged to take full personal responsibility and then the true healing process began. He apologized and I apologized and we both apologized for our part in causing pain in each other's lives. I then had to stand behind him and put my hand on his shoulder and watch him walk away. He was instructed to walk out of the building, and I wished him the best life has to offer and said out loud I release my children and trust they are fine and will continue to be fine. I then broke down crying because in my own life I was not able to do the same for my girls as I was afraid to let go. This therapy was for the gentleman, but it helped me a great deal also. It was much needed. I wrote all three of my daughters a letter when I came out of the retreat apologizing for suffocating them and not allowing them to grow.

There were various types of therapies that happened that evening some participants were given a mirror and asked to look at themselves in the mirror, others role-played not being loved, fear of death, dealing with substance abuse and dealing with mental, physical and sexual abuse. We all learned from each other and offered a loving safe environment.

## Ayahuasca #3

As in day one and two, we all gathered in the living room. The alter set again with candles, musical instruments and incense. We all looked much more relaxed and there was even giggling in the room. We were all humbled by our experience and became cheerleaders to each other.

We formed a line and when it was my turn, I knelt down but before I held the bowl of ayahuasca the shaman blew rape (a finely ground tobacco) in my nose. I then held the bowl of ayahuasca and asked, "Who am I?" I drank ayahuasca and went to my spot, grabbed my bucket, blindfolded myself and waited in a sitting position.

I then heard Mama Ayahuasca say to me "Peel of your mask." I began to peel off my mask and turned into a praying mantis and I said "Eww, why a bug?" and she said, "If you don't like it change it." I continued to peel of my layers of masks. Then I got distracted with the music that was being played I asked, "What's that eerie music?" and she said "That's not for you—others in the room need to hear that music to heal. Continue to peel." When I finally peeled the last layer off, I was a ray of white light.

She told me, "You see, that's what you are a ray of pure white light." She then took me to a higher dimension and I saw family members who were deceased. She would show me their face so I knew who they were and then they would peel their masks off and turn to pure white light and shoot up into the universe. Then we came back to earth and I saw family members here who also peeled off their masks and became pure white light and also shot up into the universe. She said, "We are all one."

The rest of the night I just continued to yawn like the lion king, I could not control it. She said, "I am healing your emotional scars with each inhalation I give you unconditional love and with each exhalation I release your emotional scars." We stayed in the living room until three or four in the morning and then most of us went back to our rooms to sleep. That night I received so many messages including writing this book and continuing to help people combining both Eastern and Western practices.

## Retreat Day 4

### Kambo #3

I was not looking forward to this. I was wiped out, it was so challenging, but I did as Mama Ayahuasca instructed me to. I drank my two liters of water and lined up with my vomit bucket in hand. When it was my turn, I sat in the chair focused on the tree and the assistant asked me, "Do you know why I ask you to focus on something?" I said, "No not really." He said, "When you have clear focus you have clear direction in life. Kambo is not only healing your physical body, but it is teaching you the importance of staying focused in life and not getting caught up in things that don't serve you." He then lit the incense stick and got some kambo and asked, "Are you ready?" I answered in a very secure voice "Yes I am." He then burned seven more spots in my arm making my cross look like a star.

Amazingly this time around I still purged but it was not as forceful or violent as day one or two and it was tolerable. I focused on the tree and on my life and on my goals, and it was a transformative experience. When I was done, I did not go to my room to sleep I actually stayed in the garden and had wonderful conversations with some of the participants. We all shared why we were there and how humbling and eye-opening this experience was for all of us.

## Ho'oponopono #2

Like the first time, we gathered in the room in the evening and the counselors asked us to share our experiences. Some participants were very happy, others not so. Most participants had incredible experiences and were very grateful to be there.

There were a couple of participants who said they did not experience anything at all. No messages, no voices, no images, nothing. They were not very happy. They said all we did was throw up the whole time we were here.

The shaman and counselors asked them if they had any idea what expectations they had before coming to the retreat. Some answered, "I wanted to hear from my loved one that died." Others said, "I wanted to talk to God." Others said, "I wanted to feel better." The shaman replied, "You see, with ayahuasca you have to drop your expectations and let go. If you resist you will not experience anything. She said ayahuasca is unpredictable, she gives you what you need not what you want. She encouraged them to give themselves some time and come back in six months. She said ayahuasca would continue to work in them during this time.

## What Did I Take Away from This Life-Changing Experience?

For the first time in my life I felt a sense of universal love and I was shown a road map that really allowed me to make a radical shift in my life. During my conversations with Ayahuasca and God I was shown very vibrant beautiful colors, many geometric images and spoke in a different language that I have never heard of in this life. I connected with my loved ones and got a sense of what it's like having pure peace.

A few weeks after this life-changing experience I quit my job in California and moved to Arizona without having a new job in place or even a home. It's like I had previously had this blindfold on and had lost touch with myself and my dharma. On the retreat, I received many messages and formed a clear picture of what I am supposed to be doing. I can say for me it was a true eye-opening experience. I faced my fears head-on and started a whole new life with a whole new perspective. I have a great sense of gratitude for this wonderful experience, and for my life.

I accepted the fact that I need to be less stringent with my daughters I need to let them live their lives and learn from their mistakes as I did. I cannot protect them from every harmful experience, and I cannot continue to feel guilty for not being with them all the time because I had to work. I did the best I could.

## Biggest Lesson for Me

I honestly thought my love for my daughters and husband was unconditional pure love, but I realized I am, or was, a hypocrite. Why do I say this? Because unconditional love expects nothing in return and I did. I expected my daughters to be good girls get good grades be successful and of course follow all my advice. With my husband, I never asked what he wanted—I just assumed he wanted what I wanted and never asked about his needs. I assumed my decisions were best for everyone. Now I know I caused great harm and I intend to fix the problem I created. I also forgive myself for I did not know any better and only repeated what I was taught.

~

# Steps I Have Taken Since Returning from My Ayahuasca Experience:

- I stopped listening to music that has no meaning and does not feed my soul.

- I am learning how to express my feelings and stop suppressing them because I know firsthand, they only cause illness.

- I stopped watching TV shows that generate fear or are not helping me grow as an individual.

- I started incorporating breathing exercises. I remember Ayahuasca telling me with every inhalation I give you unconditional love with every exhalation I take away all your emotional trauma and pain.

- I practice paying attention to my body and acknowledging how I feel. I look at what I eat and how I exercise and most important how I talk about myself.

- I schedule time to do things I enjoy more frequently. I continue to spend time with people who have the same interest as I do.

- I continue to work with spiritual healing energy and workshops, using the law of attraction and vibration, music and sound therapy, and color therapy.

- I started practicing yoga at home and continue to meditate.

- I can honestly say I always knew there was a higher being, light source, God and now I feel like I was honored to have had a conversation with God and find true peace. I feel so blessed to be part of this wonderful life.

~

# APPENDICES

~

## Chapter 1 Exercises – Finding Peace

Some ideas to help you experiment with different types of meditation.

1.  **Sitting meditation.** Find a comfortable position in a half-lotus, lotus or kneeling position. You may use a pillow or sit in a chair. Let your hands relax in your lap. Now set your intention for your meditation today. Count your breaths, breathe in through your nose and out through your mouth, and repeat seven times. Start with five minutes a day, working up to twenty minutes a day. If your mind starts wandering, acknowledge your thoughts and feelings and refocus on your breathing.

2.  **Walking meditation.** Find a safe relaxing environment; for example, a park, the beach, or even your backyard. Set your intention and begin breathing in through your nose and out through your mouth as you begin walking. Pay attention to your feet. The steps should be more deliberate than your usual walking. If you feel any soreness or tightness, acknowledge it and try to relax. Start with fifteen minutes, working up to thirty minutes

3. **Guided meditation.** Search online to find one that resonates with you—there are lots!

4. **Create an altar.** This is your sacred space. You can have candles, incense, images, crystals, or anything that allows you to connect and relax. This is your personal space, so feel free to create it to align with your own beliefs.

5. **Take time to reflect.** Which meditation did you enjoy the most and why?

_____

_____

_____

6. **Download an app.** There are some fantastic options available. The ones I use for meditation include Omvana and Calm.

Your Reflections _____

_____

_____

_____

_____

_____

_____

# APPENDICES

---

---

---

---

---

---

---

---

---

---

---

---

---

---

---

---

# Chapter 2 Exercises – Complete Control

Here are some everyday activities you can start incorporating in your daily routine to reduce stress and keep your emotions under control.

1. Disconnect for one day, no electrical devices.

2. Sign up for and attend a yoga, tai chi or Qigong class.

3. Go for a walk in the park or along the beach.

4. Practice the grounding exercise discussed in this book.

5. Sign up for a craniosacral therapy.

6. Talk about your feelings. I can't emphasize this enough.

7. Practice forgiveness, not for them but for you.

8. Journal and release any emotions you might be harboring.

9. Practice the tapping exercises discussed in this book.

*I have attended many therapeutic counselling sessions during my forty-seven years. These include hypnotherapy, biomagnetism therapy, communicating with angels, acupuncture, craniosacral therapy, Reiki, astrology, numerology, energy healing, spirit guide readings, transformational therapy, and plant medicine healing using ho'oponopono therapy. I share this with you because you might need to experiment with different therapies until you find what is best for you.*

Your Reflections _____

_____

# APPENDICES

_____

_____

_____

_____

_____

_____

_____

_____

_____

_____

_____

_____

_____

_____

_____

_____

_____

# Chapter 3 Exercises – Energy Boost

Some simple steps to balancing work, life, and a healthy lifestyle.

1. Start an exercise routine. It is well-known that exercise releases endorphins that help to decrease stress. To help you keep track you can download an app such as MyFitnessPal or Pacer, to name a few.

2. Create healthy meal recipes that include whole grains, lean protein, fruits, and vegetables of the full color spectrum. Incorporate meal prepping for lunch instead of eating out.

3. Take your daily multivitamin and supplements, and include herbal teas. Drink eight cups of water per day.

4. Practice daily gratitude. Be thankful for what you have. Dump negative thinking. Harboring negative emotions can lead to disease and illness, so be aware of your negative thinking and dump it. Let it go. Forgive and forget. This can be very difficult to do, but remember, you are doing this for you, not for them. Imagine how good your life will be when you stop carrying that burden.

5. Unwind using meditation, yoga, tai chi, soak in the tub or read a good book. Schedule regular time walking in nature—in the park, at the beach, hiking, or by a river.

6. Aim for seven to eight hours of quality sleep every night.

7. Remember to laugh, laugh, and laugh. Find ways to smile more and laugh more. Spend time with people who bring out the best in you.

# APPENDICES

Your Reflections _____

_____

_____

_____

_____

_____

_____

_____

_____

_____

_____

_____

_____

_____

_____

_____

# Chapter 4 Exercises – Abundance Now

Here are some simple ways you can practice daily gratitude.

1. Take a minute right now to journal five great things that happened today. Acknowledge your emotions as your write and then read back what you are grateful for. This happy feeling is the feeling you should have when you set your intentions.

2. Start a daily gratitude list. Read it every morning and every night. Keep your journal at your bedside so you don't forget a day. Practice makes perfect.

3. If you feel like complaining, give yourself five minutes to let it out and then let it go. Please don't go to bed upset or angry. Let it go. Over time these emotions can bring on illness, so let's prevent them.

4. Remember to say please and thank you—it goes a long way. Give it a try.

5. When you are having a bad day, stop complaining and start thinking about all the good things you have going on in your life. My belief is "like attracts like." I have seen firsthand what happens when people spend all their time and energy complaining—they attract more obstacles to their lives. It's a vicious cycle.

Your Reflections _____

_____

_____

_____

# APPENDICES

## Chapter 5 Exercises – Success Patterns

### Goal worksheet

**Start Date:** _____        **End Date:** _____

My goal is:

_____

_____

_____

My goal is important to me because:

_____

_____

_____

_____

What three steps will I take today to reach my goal:

1. _____

_____

_____

2. _____

_____

_____

3. _____

_____

_____

What are some limiting beliefs I have that might prevent me from reaching my goal:

_____

_____

_____

How will I feel if I don't reach my goal because of my limiting beliefs?

_____

_____

_____

# HELP YOURSELF...

Who can I reach out to for support and how can they help me?

Your Reflections _____

_____

_____

_____

_____

_____

_____

_____

_____

_____

_____

_____

_____

_____

_____

_____

# Chapter 6 Exercises – Vision to Reality

Try these ideas to help you visualize and manifest what you want in life.

1.  Create a vision board using magazine pictures, phrases, and articles. I've hung my vision board on the wall in my bedroom next to my bed. It's the first thing I see when I wake up and the last thing I see when I go to bed.

2.  Work on creative projects. Dedicate thirty minutes three to four times a week to work on a project. Work on something that brings you joy.

3.  Spend time in nature either in a park, at the beach, or in the mountains. This is so important. We get so caught up in our hectic lives and we need to replenish by reconnecting to nature. This will help us think outside the box and spark creative thinking skills.

4.  Set time aside to travel. Go somewhere unfamiliar to you. Network, meet new people, try different foods, go sightseeing. This will also get your creative flow going.

5.  At least two or three times a week, set time aside to be by yourself. Close your eyes and visualize what you want (your goal). As you visualize, bring in all positive emotions relating to this goal as if you have already accomplished it. This is so important. This is the feeling you want to have when you set new goals.

6.  If you are having a difficult day at work or at home, take a couple of minutes out and take a few slow deep breaths. You can also practice the tapping exercises discussed in the book.

HELP YOURSELF...

Your Reflections _____

_____

_____

_____

_____

_____

_____

_____

_____

_____

_____

_____

_____

_____

_____

_____

# Chapter 7 Exercises – Ultimate Balance

Here's how to balance each of your seven chakras.

1.  Root chakra—walk around barefoot, practice stretching exercises and dance.
    * daily affirmation: "I am safe"
    * foods: red fruits and vegetables, such as red apples, strawberries, tomatoes, raspberries and cherries
    * essential oil: clove
    * meditation chant: "LAM"
    * yoga pose: Tree Pose

2.  Sacral chakra—take a long bath with Epsom salt, baking soda and Himalayan salt.
    * daily affirmation: "I am creative and adaptable"
    * foods: orange fruits and vegetables, such as mangos, carrots, oranges, apricots and papaya
    * essential oil: sandalwood
    * meditation chant: "VAM"
    * yoga pose: Goddess Pose

3.  Solar plexus chakra—spend some time in the sun, do things that build your self-esteem and confidence.
    * daily affirmation: "I can do anything I set my mind to"
    * foods: yellow fruits and vegetables, such as yellow bell pepper, squash, lemons and pineapple
    * essential oil: lemon
    * meditation chant: "RAM"
    * yoga pose: Boat Pose

4.  Heart chakra—work on fulfilling your dreams and desires.
    * daily affirmation: "I am loving and lovable"
    * foods: green colored fruits and vegetables such as green apples, key limes, nopal (Mexican cactus), avocados, dark leafy green vegetables

- essential oil: rose
- meditation chant: "YAM"
- yoga pose: Camel Pose

5.  Throat chakra—sing your heart out, practice saying "no".
    - daily affirmation: "I know my truth and I share it"
    - foods: blueberries
    - essential oil: lavender or sage
    - meditation chant: "HAM"
    - yoga pose: Supported Shoulder stand

6.  Third eye chakra—practice fasting.
    - daily affirmation, "I am intuitive and follow my inner guidance"
    - foods: herbal teas, blueberries, grapes, blackberries and plums
    - essential oil: patchouli
    - meditation chant: "OM"
    - yoga pose: Easy Pose

7.  Crown chakra—meditate, include quiet time in your daily schedule.
    - daily affirmation: "I am intelligent and aware"
    - foods: herbal teas, elderberries and grapes
    - essential oil: frankincense
    - meditation chant: "OM"
    - yoga pose: Corpse Pose

Your Reflections _____

_____

_____

_____

# APPENDICES

_____

_____

_____

_____

_____

_____

_____

_____

_____

_____

_____

_____

_____

_____

_____

_____

# Chapter 8 Exercises – Beyond Guilt

Activities you can incorporate in your daily life to remove feelings of guilt.

1.  Listen to happy songs and sing along.

2.  Go for a massage, manicure, or pedicure. Or even better, sign up for craniosacral massage, biomagnetism, or acupuncture therapies.

3.  Got to the movies or go dancing.

4.  Surround yourself with people who love you and support you.

5.  Go on vacation or a road trip.

6.  Meet a friend for coffee or lunch.

7.  Practice tapping exercises and daily affirmations to eliminate guilt, stress, and anxiety.

Your Reflections _____

_____

_____

_____

_____

_____

_____

# APPENDICES

---

---

---

---

---

---

---

---

---

---

---

---

---

---

---

---

---

# Chapter 9 Exercises – Unlocking Communication

Try these simple ways to enhance your communication skills.

1. Unfollow people on social media who don't inspire you.

2. Have a phone-free night.

3. Unsubscribe from email marketing.

4. Clean out your inbox. Once I had 90,000 emails at one time. This was so exhausting! Never again.

5. Say goodbye to toxic people in your life.

6. Have you noticed any "bad" communication habits? If so, what can you do to catch yourself and break it?

7. What are some things you can do to ensure you are really communicating well with someone?

8. We are not always clear about saying "no." This was difficult for me. I am a people pleaser. I had to remind myself I have the right to say "no." This prevents a lot of stress and burnout in my life. I encourage you to try it.

Your Reflections _____

_____

_____

_____

_____

# APPENDICES

_____

_____

_____

_____

_____

_____

_____

_____

_____

_____

_____

_____

_____

_____

_____

_____

_____

_____

# Chapter 10 Exercises – Do Your Own Thing

Activities to awaken your God-given gifts.

1. What is on your bucket list? What brings you joy? What brings you happiness? Imagine that time and money are not barriers. Write them down and see yourself accomplishing your list. How do you feel? What steps can you start taking today that will get you closer to accomplishing your goals and desires. Most importantly, be yourself. Be true to yourself, you don't have to impress anyone, and your uniqueness is what makes you shine. So, share it with the world, don't be shy.

**Daily affirmation: "I create my future. I am the author of my life."**

2. Set time aside to read and work on your hobbies, your God-given talents. Learn to cultivate them. I enjoy listening to Tony Robbins and Oprah Winfrey for my dose of daily motivation. Give of yourself, share your talents. When we share our talents and give of our time, it feels good to be of service to someone else. This can be in the form of coaching, or just lending an ear. Remember, pay it forward.

**Daily affirmation: "I am creative and have a lot to contribute. Every day I discover new hidden talents about myself and I am ready to share them with the world."**

3. What do you see yourself doing to have less stress? Does this include going back to school for more training, changing jobs, moving up in your current job, or cutting back to part time and starting a side business, to share your talents with others?

**Daily affirmation: "I do what I love on a daily basis."**

4.  Set financial goals to allow you to get closer to accomplishing your life goals and desires. This includes setting up a budget sheet to write down what comes in and what goes out. What can you cut back on to help you save? Set up direct deposit and pay yourself first. Set up auto payments to avoid any late fees. Look for cheaper insurance. Shop around. It takes work, but it's worth it. When I am planning my trips, I plan them out for a year. I figure out how much money I will need, and I then divide it by twelve. This gives me a clear picture of how much I need to save each month to reach that goal. You can do the same to pay down debt. It is a very good feeling when you have money set aside to do the things you love and enjoy. Don't forget your emergency fund. This is very important. The recommendation is that you have a least three months of all your bills set aside, this includes your mortgage.

**Daily affirmation: "I am financially prosperous. I generate income from known and unknown sources."**

5.  Find a mentor. Who do you admire? If you can close your eyes and picture your mentor, what is his/her daily routine? What steps does he/she take to succeed? Read about the mentor prospect, and if you can take a seminar, sign up. Of course, you must be willing to do the work just like he or she did, with a clear focus. We are constantly learning and evolving.

**Daily affirmation: "When I need help, I always attract successful, caring and generous mentors into my life who guide me and show me how to grow both personally and professionally."**

6.  Choose your circle. Remember to surround yourself with people who bring out the best in you, people you can learn from, people who have walked the path you are starting. These days, with social media, this has become easier.

**Daily affirmation: "I am surrounded by positive, inspirational and supportive people who believe in me and I trust my inspiration and trust people who respect me."**

Your Reflections _____

_____

_____

_____

_____

_____

_____

_____

_____

_____

_____

_____

_____

# Chapter 11 Exercises – Heal Yourself

Here are some simple ideas to help you practice self-care.

1.  Put yourself first. Learn to love yourself first. Assess and address your needs. Do something for yourself.

2.  Take a nap, meditate, practice acupressure on yourself, practice daily breathing exercises.

3.  Treat yourself to a spa day, take a day off, schedule a weekend getaway or mini vacation.

4.  Do something that energizes your body. Stretch, swim, go for a walk in the park, ride your bike, any physical activity you enjoy.

5.  Take regular breaks and avoid working through lunch.

6.  Research and try some of the healing therapies discussed in this chapter.

Your Reflections _____

_____

_____

_____

_____

_____

_____

# HELP YOURSELF...

# ABOUT THE AUTHOR

~

Lillian was raised by a single mother in Los Angeles, California, along with her brother and sister. Her mother immigrated from Mexico and worked as a seamstress. She instilled in Lillian the value of getting an education. Lillian's mother worked diligently and saved up to open her own business, becoming a business owner at the age of twenty-one.

At the age of sixteen, Lillian dropped out of high school and this upset her mother. She had hoped Lillian would finish her education because she herself was only able to finish sixth grade because her family was poor, and she needed to work and contribute to the household. She gave Lillian two options: to return to school or get a job. Lillian chose to get a job, but little did she know her mother was going to send her to Idaho for the summer to work with the migrant workers. Lillian packed her bags and went off to Idaho to pick cherries, apples, nectarines, and apricots. This was a very difficult job. She woke up at four o'clock in the morning, packed burritos for lunch, and went to work from sunup to sundown. She lived there for three months, worked full time, paid bills and rent, and had very little money left as she was only paid the minimum wage. This was life changing for Lillian as she was unaware of how difficult life was without an education and for immigrants.

When she returned home, her mother asked her, "Well, what did you think? You know you are a citizen of the United States and you are blessed to have so many choices and opportunities. You can choose to work with your hands or get educated and work with your brain. The people you were working with were undocumented and have limited choices. They wish they had the opportunities you have, yet you choose to waste them." Lillian eagerly replied, "No, Mom, I am ready to go back to school." Lillian went back to school, received her GED, a couple months later her high school diploma, and shortly after she became a certified nursing assistant at the age of seventeen. Lillian's Aunt Silvia and Aunt Mirin also had a big impact on Lillian's childhood, teaching her to look at the challenges and struggles of life as opportunity for learning and growth.

Lillian has been in the nursing field for thirty years. She started as a certified nursing assistant at the age of seventeen, then went on to pursue her licensed vocational nurse, associates, bachelors, and master's degrees in nursing. She is currently a family nurse practitioner and a board-certified doctor of holistic health. She is also a Reiki master and an energy healer. Lillian has always had a passion for learning and helping others. She has worked in home health, med-surg, subacute, kidney liver transplant, mother baby, emergency room, and care management of diabetic patients. She also owned and operated two assisted living homes in Arizona. She has studied homeopathy, herbology, biomagnetism, and continues to attend seminars and classes to keep expanding her knowledge.

Lillian has many things for which to be grateful in her life. She has a loving husband, three beautiful, intelligent daughters and three wonderful grandchildren.

Lillian's passion is to open a wellness center that combines Eastern and Western healing. The goal with the wellness center and this book is to help others to gain the knowledge required to practice self-care and self-healing. With so many years in the health care profession, Lillian has seen the toll it takes on nurses and health-care providers, affecting their health and emotional well-being. In her wellness center, she will teach people how to heal themselves and others. This is the answer for which she was waiting.

For now, Lillian has put together this book to share her practices with all of you in the hopes of teaching you how to heal yourself. Lillian believes if we are healthy and happy, then we will transmit that energy to our patients, clients, family, friends, and pets.

Dr. Lillian Gonzalez, BCDHH, FNP, MSN, Reiki Master,
Energy Healer and Author
Synergy Holistic Care & Wellness LLC

Website: synergyhcw.com

Email: synergyhcw@gmail.com
Facebook: @synergyhcw
Instagram: @synergy_holisticcare_wellness

# OFFER 1

# HALF-DAY SELF-CARE WORKSHOP FOR HEALTH-CARE PROFESSIONALS

~

**H**alf-day workshops for health-care providers that are delivered in your workplace to individuals or small groups. The workshop will show you why self-care is essential for medical professionals and share simple and effective techniques that you can implement into your everyday life. The topics covered include:

1. An honest review of how you currently take care of yourself
2. Uncover the reasons why nurses experience burnout
3. Practical and effective techniques to help you avoid nursing burnout
4. Informative discussion of non-conventional healing therapies
5. Simple self-care exercises to implement to assist you in your healing journey

To find out more contact:

Dr. Lillian Gonzalez, BCDHH, FNP, MSN, Reiki Master,
Energy Healer and Author

Synergy Holistic Care & Wellness LLC
Phone 323-286-5899

Website: synergyhcw.com
Email: synergyhcw@gmail.com
Facebook: @synergyhcw
Instagram: @synergy_holisticcare_wellness

## OFFER 2

# ONLINE SELF-CARE LEARNING COURSE FOR HEALTH-CARE PROFESSIONALS

~

An online learning program that can be completed at your own pace from the comfort of your home. The program is full of easy to follow tips and techniques for health-care professionals to help you practice self-care in your daily life. The modules covered include:

1. An honest review of how you currently take care of yourself
2. Uncover the reasons why nurses experience burnout
3. Practical and effective techniques to help you avoid nursing burnout
4. Informative discussion of non-conventional healing therapies
5. Simple self-care exercises to implement to assist you in your healing journey

**To find out more contact:**

Dr. Lillian Gonzalez, BCDHH, FNP, MSN, Reiki Master, Energy Healer and Author

Synergy Holistic Care & Wellness LLC
Phone 323-286-5899

Website: synergyhcw.com
Email: synergyhcw@gmail.com
Facebook: @synergyhcw
Instagram: @synergy_holisticcare_wellness

# OFFER 3

# HOLISTIC HEALTH ASSESSMENT AND COACHING

~

**H**olistic health practitioners treat the whole person, not just individual parts, to enhance your overall health. It involves identifying and treating the cause of the condition, rather than only alleviating the symptoms. Holistic health treatments can help with many common conditions such as chronic fatigue, body aches, diabetes, irritable bowel syndrome, obesity, depression, anxiety and stress to name a few.

- Your initial assessment includes a review of your existing physical, mental, emotional, and spiritual well-being.
- From there we will devise a strategy to treat any areas of concern.
- Your plan will include a combination of complementary and alternative approaches that will improve your health and well-being in both the short and long term.

**To schedule your consultation contact:**

Dr. Lillian Gonzalez, BCDHH, FNP, MSN, Reiki Master, Energy Healer and Author

Synergy Holistic Care & Wellness LLC
Phone 323-286-5899

Website: synergyhcw.com
Email: synergyhcw@gmail.com
Facebook: @synergyhcw
Instagram: @synergy_holisticcare_wellness

www.ingramcontent.com/pod-product-compliance
Lightning Source LLC
Chambersburg PA
CBHW022054020426
42335CB00012B/689